THE MOMMY MAKEOVER

How Real Moms Reclaim Confidence, Connection, and Their Reflection

By Michael R. Burgdorf, MD, MPH

Award-Winning, Board-Certified Plastic Surgeon
Founder of Music City Plastic Surgery
www.musiccityplasticsurgery.com
307 Southgate Court, Suite 100, Brentwood, TN 37027

Published by Music City Media Group.

For the mothers who carried life,
loved deeply,
sacrificed quietly—
and are ready to see themselves again.

TABLE OF CONTENTS

A Letter to the Mom Reading This Book

If you're holding this book, there's a good chance you've had a moment with a mirror.

Not a long moment.

Just a quick pause.

Maybe while getting dressed.
Maybe after a shower.
Maybe when trying on clothes that used to fit differently.

And somewhere in that moment, a quiet thought appeared:

"Is this really my body now?"

If that thought has ever crossed your mind, I want you to know something right away.

You are not alone.

Over the years, thousands of women have sat across from me in my office and shared that same feeling—sometimes in words, sometimes in silence.

They come in carrying many things:

Love for their children.
Gratitude for their families.
Pride in what their bodies accomplished.

But often they are also carrying something else.

A quiet sense that somewhere along the way, a part of themselves got lost.

Not because motherhood diminished them.

But because motherhood asked so much of them.

Pregnancy stretches the body in extraordinary ways.
Breastfeeding changes the breasts.
The abdomen expands to make room for new life.

These changes are not signs of failure.

They are signs of something remarkable.

But that doesn't mean you're wrong for wondering whether your body could feel strong, comfortable, or familiar again.

Wanting to feel confident in your body is not vanity.

It's human.

And it's especially understandable for women who have spent years caring for everyone else first.

This book is not about chasing perfection.

It's about understanding what pregnancy actually changes in the body—and what options exist if you want to restore parts of what changed.

Along the way, you'll meet other women who have walked this journey.

You'll learn the truth about procedures, recovery, and expectations.

And most importantly, you'll hear something many moms have never been told clearly enough:

Your body didn't fail you.

It carried your children.

Whatever path you ultimately choose—whether that includes surgery, lifestyle changes, or simply a new understanding of your body—I hope this book helps you see yourself with greater clarity and compassion.

Because the woman you are today deserves to feel seen.

And she deserves to feel at home in her own reflection again.

With respect and gratitude,

Michael R. Burgdorf, MD, MPH

The Mommy Makeover Promise

A note about how I approach this work—and what you deserve as a patient.

If you're reading this book, you may be wondering whether restoring parts of your body after pregnancy is the right step for you.

Before we go any further, I want to make a few promises.

These are the same principles I bring into every consultation room and every operating room.

I Promise to Tell You the Truth

Not every concern requires surgery.

Not every procedure is the right solution for every patient.

My responsibility as a surgeon is not to sell procedures—it is to help you understand what is truly possible and what is not.

Sometimes the most ethical recommendation is to wait.

Sometimes it is to choose a smaller solution.

And sometimes surgery truly can restore something meaningful.

I Promise That Natural Results Matter More Than Dramatic Ones

The best plastic surgery should never look like plastic surgery.

My goal is never to create a different person.

It is to restore balance so that when someone sees you, they simply think:

"You look amazing."

Not:

"You look like you had surgery."

I Promise That Safety Comes First

Beautiful results mean nothing if they are not achieved safely with you available to enjoy the results. I understand you are a mom whose family needs you.

Every surgical decision should prioritize:

- your health
- your healing
- your long-term wellbeing

A responsible surgeon respects the body's limits.

I Promise That Your Confidence Matters More Than Perfection

No surgical procedure creates perfection.

But restoring your body's structure can help many women feel stronger, more comfortable, and more confident.

The goal is not flawlessness.

The goal is alignment between how you feel inside and how you move through the world.

I Promise to Respect Your Journey of Motherhood

The women who walk through my doors are not simply patients.

They are mothers.

Women who grew life inside, sacrificed deeply, and spent years putting others first.

If part of your journey now includes restoring parts of your body, that decision deserves compassion—not judgment.

And One Final Promise

Whatever path you choose after reading this book—whether it includes surgery or not—I hope you walk away with one clear understanding:

Your body did not fail you.

It carried your children.

You deserve to feel at home in it again.

And I Promise, You Are Worthy of That!

For the Woman You Used to Be

There was a version of you
who moved through the world differently.

Before the schedules.
Before the responsibilities.
Before your body became a place others depended on.

She is not gone.

She is still here—
woven into everything you've carried,
everything you've given,
everything you've become.

This book is not about going back to her.

It's about recognizing that
she never really left.

As you turn these pages,
may you find pieces of yourself
you haven't seen in a while.

Not lost.

Just waiting.

PART I
SEEING YOURSELF AGAIN

Reclaiming Your Reflection: You Gave Life, Now Let's Give Something Back To You

Preface
The Mirror Moment

Motherhood asks everything of you—your time, your sleep, your energy, your body. During pregnancy, every choice you make is for someone else's well-being. You give up caffeine, sushi, wine, comfort, and even your own breath at times, just to protect the small life inside you. And you do it willingly.

You expect the fatigue, the cravings, the stretching. What most women don't expect is the quiet grief that comes later—months after the sleepless nights fade, when you finally catch a glimpse of yourself in the mirror and whisper, "What happened to me?"

In that instant, it can feel like there were two births that day: your child, and a new version of you—the one wearing the "mom body" you never met before.

Maybe you first saw her in a passing reflection, or maybe your toddler brought her into focus with a comment far too honest to ignore: "Mommy, why is your belly still big?" They mean no harm. But the sting is real.

Many mothers carry that quiet ache for years—the tug between gratitude for what their bodies have done and the discomfort of no longer recognizing the person in the mirror. They push it aside with diets, workouts, and "supermom" expectations, pretending it doesn't bother them. But it does.

This book is written for that woman—the one who loves her children deeply but misses herself profoundly.

My hope is that within these pages you'll discover what so many of my patients have found: that your beauty and confidence were never lost—only hidden. Waiting, patiently, to be uncovered.

Together, we'll talk honestly about what happens to your body and your heart after childbirth. We'll separate myths from medicine, guilt from grace. And along the way, I'll invite you to participate in simple reflections that help you reconnect with yourself again.

Let's begin with a note—not to your children, but to yourself.

The Reflection Letter:

Write a letter to your "before-kids" self. Tell her what she's about to accomplish, what she'll endure, and how strong she'll become. Remind her that beauty doesn't disappear—it evolves. Tell her she's still in there, waiting to be seen again.

You don't have to bounce back. You just have to come back—to you.

CHAPTER 1

The Body That Doesn't Feel Like Mine Anymore

The Moment She Looked in the Mirror

I've lost count of how many times I've stood beside a woman looking at her reflection after surgery—tears gathering, shoulders lifting, voice trembling.

"I feel like myself again," she says.
Not "I look younger." Not "I finally fit in these jeans." Just myself again.

That simple phrase has stopped me in my tracks more times than any before-and-after photo ever could.

Early in my career, I inherently understood that plastic surgery was more than just technique— the perfect incision, the right symmetry. While I appreciate the precision of technique, the underlying impact on life is what spoke to my soul when choosing my career in plastic surgery. And the longer I've done this work, the more I've realized that what's really being repaired isn't just skin or muscle. It's identity. And oftentimes, it's relationships—with a spouse, with children, and most importantly, with self.

I call it the **ripple effect** of plastic surgery. When a woman restores her confidence, that energy radiates outward. I've seen marriages reconnect, laughter return to homes, and women show up in their lives with a presence they thought they'd lost forever.

When Your Reflection Doesn't Match Your Reality

Every mom I meet has her own version of **the mirror moment**. Some say, "I still look six months pregnant." Others tug at loose skin or whisper about breasts that no longer sit where they once did.

But what connects them all is the same deep dissonance: *the body doesn't feel like home anymore.*

You might eat well, exercise, and take care of everyone around you — yet somehow, the reflection looking back feels foreign. You know who you are inside, but your body doesn't seem to have gotten the message.

That disconnect isn't about vanity; it's about alignment. When the person you *feel* you are inside doesn't match what you *see* outside, it can affect everything — confidence, intimacy, even energy. And that misalignment ripples beyond you, shaping the tone of your home, your relationships, your joy. I've had moms tell me they wouldn't dare go to the pool or take the kids on a beach vacation with "the way I look." It becomes harder to show up fully in life when you're quietly fighting yourself.

Medically, this is not a moral failure—it's structure. After pregnancy, your abdominal wall — the core muscles that once pulled everything tight — can separate. That condition, called **diastasis recti**, isn't something you can "crunch" away. Add stretched skin, hormonal shifts, and natural fat redistribution, and your once-familiar shape starts to feel like a stranger's.

And yet society sends mothers the same message, over and over again: *Just work harder.* The "bounce back" myth tells you that if you really cared, you'd somehow find the energy to eat clean, train intensely, and ignore the exhaustion. It whispers that you're supposed to love your "battle scars" and that wanting change means you're ungrateful.

That message is wrong — and it's cruel.

Because what's actually happening to your body is biology, not failure.

Understanding What Really Happened (and How to Begin Healing)

The first step toward healing is grace.

You didn't fail your body. Your body succeeded — spectacularly.

It created life, supported it, nourished it. That takes an enormous physical toll that no diet or gym routine can ever fully reverse. As my wife would remind me after each of our four children were born, "something breaks with each pregnancy."

Your body deserves respect—and, if you choose, restoration.

Understanding the "why" behind the changes is the first step toward reclaiming yourself:

- **Your muscles stretched** to make room for a growing baby — sometimes separating at the midline (diastasis recti).

- **Your skin expanded** beyond its original elasticity, leaving laxity that can't retract on its own. In my office, we talk a lot about the "overstretched rubber-band phenomenon."
- **Your hormones shifted**, altering how and where your body stores fat.
- **Your posture adapted** for months — which can make your core feel weaker even after recovery.

Knowing these facts often lifts the fog of self-blame.

From there, the path forward becomes clearer — and personalized.

Some women heal through focused exercise and time. Others benefit from physical therapy, or non-surgical treatments that tighten skin or contour stubborn areas. And for those whose anatomy simply can't return to its pre-pregnancy structure without help, **surgical repair** — a tummy tuck, breast lift, labiaplasty, or combined "Mommy Makeover" —becomes the physical and emotional reset they've longed for.

The moment I see that shift in a patient — when she stands taller, eyes bright, a deep exhale she didn't know she was holding — it's not about "fixing" her. It's about restoring alignment between how she feels and what she sees.

That's what healing looks like.
Not chasing perfection — *coming home* to yourself again.

A Mommy Makeover isn't about vanity—it's about visibility. It's about helping women reconnect with the version of themselves that motherhood often asks them to forget.

As a husband, father, and surgeon, I've seen how easily mothers disappear behind the title of "Mom."
Not all at once—but gradually, quietly, without announcement.

This book is my attempt to hold up a mirror—
not just to your reflection, but to your worth.

Whether you ever have surgery or not, you deserve to feel confident, connected, and whole.

You gave life.
Now it's time to give something back to you.

And maybe, as you begin, you'll recognize someone you haven't seen in a while.

Your Mirror Truth Exercise

This next step isn't about surgery. It's about self-awareness.

Tonight, find a quiet moment and stand before the mirror—not as a critic, but as a witness. Not the rushed glance you give yourself while brushing your teeth — a deliberate pause.

Look at your reflection and, for once, don't analyze. Just *notice.*

Then, write down:

1. **Three ways your body has served you**. (It carried you through something extraordinary — maybe childbirth, maybe something else entirely.) Or write down 3 ways Motherhood has strengthened you.
2. **One part of yourself** — physical, emotional, or spiritual — that you'd like to reconnect with this year.
3. **One small action** you can take this week to begin that reconnection.

This isn't about judgment. It's about compassion.

Because before any physical transformation happens, an emotional one must begin — the moment you decide to see yourself not as broken, but as *becoming.*

Closing Reflection

You gave life. You sacrificed your body, your time, your sleep, your energy — often without a second thought.
Now, for the first time in a long time, it's okay to think about *you.*

This chapter isn't your destination.
It's the door opening — the moment you take your reflection back from everything that's claimed it.
And when you do, I promise — the woman staring back will finally feel familiar again.

CHAPTER 2
The Myths of the "Bounce Back"

The phrase shows up everywhere—magazines, podcasts, even well-meaning friends: "She bounced back so fast after the baby!" It's said as praise, but what it really does is plant a quiet seed of pressure.

I remember a patient named Sarah who came to see me nine months after giving birth to her second child. She'd lost most of her pregnancy weight, but she said she still felt "soft" and "tired-looking." She confessed that she avoided mom groups because every conversation seemed to circle back to diet challenges or workout routines. "Everyone's competing to see who can disappear fastest," she said. "I'm still trying to catch my breath."

That's what the "bounce back" culture does—it turns recovery into a race. And motherhood was never meant to be a race.

Somewhere along the way, the miracle of what the body did became less interesting than how quickly it could erase the evidence. Social media hasn't helped. Algorithms reward transformation photos, not the months of exhaustion, healing, and hormonal chaos that happen in between. The internet loves a before-and-after; it has no patience for during.

But what if the real power isn't in bouncing back, but in building forward?

Biologically, your body isn't even designed to return to its exact pre-baby state. The hips widen, ligaments stretch, the rib cage subtly shifts, and the very architecture of your abdomen changes. You can strengthen, tone, and optimize—but "back" isn't the right direction. "Forward" is.

When I explain this to my patients, I often see relief in their faces. They've been chasing a mirage of perfection that was never realistic. The goal is restoration and balance, not reversal.

Let's talk honestly about why "bouncing back" is so alluring. It promises control in a season that feels unpredictable. Motherhood dismantles routine, privacy, and predictability—and the fitness or diet plan becomes a way to reclaim order. The problem is that when results don't match expectations, the disappointment feels personal.

You didn't fail. The promise failed you.

Here's the truth no influencer will post: most mothers' bodies need time, and sometimes help, to recover structurally.

- Separated muscles can't realign without surgical repair.

- Skin that's lost elasticity won't "tighten up" with creams or crunches.

- Hormones that supported pregnancy now shift metabolism, often causing temporary fat retention.

Your worth isn't measured by how fast you erase the evidence of giving life—it's measured by how gently you give yourself grace while you heal.

When I perform a Mommy Makeover, it isn't to make a woman "look like she never had kids." It's to help her look like she feels inside: confident, energized, and comfortable in her own skin again.

Sometimes, that means removing the reminders that don't align with how she wants to live the next chapter of her story. Sometimes it means simply teaching her that what she's seeing is normal.

If I could give every new mom one prescription, it wouldn't start in the operating room. It would start in the mirror: a daily dose of compassion, three deep breaths, and a reminder—"I'm healing, not failing."

Your Bounce Back Truth

Now I want you to try something simple. Tonight, scroll back through your photos—not the posed ones, but the candid ones from the months after giving birth. Notice what you were doing: holding, feeding, surviving, smiling through fatigue. Write down three moments that remind you of your strength. That's progress worth celebrating.

Then write one sentence that starts with: "Going forward, I want my body to help me..."—and finish it honestly. Maybe it's "...run with my kids," "...feel confident in clothes I love," or "...sleep through the night without pain." Whatever it is, that's your new direction. Not backward. Forward.

Because the truth is, the women who seem to have "bounced back" the fastest aren't necessarily happier—they're often just hiding the same insecurities everyone else has. Real confidence isn't built in comparison. It's built in compassion. And self-compassion, I've learned, is the most powerful kind of makeover there is.

MOMMY MAKEOVER MYTHS

Myth: It's been three months since my baby was born, I should have "bounced back" by now.

Reality: Each body heals in its own time. Recovery is not a race.

Myth: I need my body to just bounce back already.

Reality: Most mothers' bodies need time, and sometimes help, to recover structurally. "Building forward" can be better and healthier than just "bouncing back".

Myth: Moms don't need surgery. Diet and Exercise will help her bounce back fine.

Reality: Each mom deserves her own choice. Some bodies require more than diet and exercise to get desired results.

Myth: If I just hurry up and have surgery, all my problems will be solved.

Reality: The body needs time to heal from pregnancy and, while surgery may be a good option for some, it is not a quick fix option.

Myth: Exercise can lift and augment your breasts naturally.

Reality: Not so. You can exercise hours every day, and your breasts will still be droopy. Your pectoral muscles will be in good shape, but the size of your breasts won't change.

Myth: You can't breast-feed after a breast lift.

Reality: While this hasn't been completely proven one way or the other, the consensus is that about two-thirds of all women can breast-feed before breast surgery; about two-thirds can breast-feed afterward. It is important to choose an experienced, board-certified plastic surgeon who knows how to preserve breast function.

Myth: If you have breast implants, a mammogram can rupture them.

Reality: Unlikely to occur, unless there are capsular contractures present (see chapter 18).

Myth: Exercise will tighten your tummy and get you back to the way you were before the baby.

Reality: No amount of exercise can tighten up fibrous tissue that has been stretched by pregnancy (diastasis recti).

Myth: Rubbing creams into your abdomen and breasts will prevent stretch marks.

Reality: When the skin is stretched by the natural swelling of pregnancy and breast-feeding, the marks may fade a bit, but they are permanent, a form of scarring. The best practice is to reduce the problem by maintaining good hydration and having moderate weight gain throughout pregnancy.

Myth: If you have liposuction, you can't regain weight in that area.

Reality: Yes, you can. With large weight gain, you can actually eat through the liposuction.

Myth: A Mommy Makeover isn't safe.

Reality: All surgery has some risk, but a Mommy Makeover is very safe when performed by an experienced, board-certified plastic surgeon.

Myth: You will look plastic or fake after the surgery.

Reality: A skilled surgeon will give you natural-looking results. Subtlety is key.

Myth: Everybody will know I had surgery.

Reality: Only if you tell them—which I hope you do and refer them to me as patients.

Myth: My husband just won't understand.

Reality: You don't know that until you talk about it. He may surprise you and be very supportive—that has been my experience with my patients over the years.

Myth: I can't afford it.

Reality: Yes, a Mommy Makeover costs real money and is not covered by insurance. Think of it as an investment in yourself.

Myth: I'm not worth it.

Reality: *Yes, you are.*

Myth: I'm not ready to have such confidence.

Reality: Look out, world!

Myth: I'll never get my body back to what it was before my baby.

Reality: You will be surprised how your Mommy Makeover will impact you, your body, and relationships, even making them better than before.

CHAPTER 3

Redefining the Mommy Makeover

When most people hear the phrase "Mommy Makeover," they picture a glossy ad, a dramatic before-and-after photo, or a celebrity headline. But that's not what I see.

What I see are women uncovering the version of themselves they thought had disappeared—the confident, radiant woman whose reflection once matched how she felt inside. *A Mommy Makeover isn't about becoming someone new. It's about uncovering who you've been all along.*

The phrase itself can feel intimidating, even indulgent. For some women, it sounds commercialized or self-centered, a luxury reserved for others. I've had patients whisper it under their breath in consultations, as if saying it out loud might make them sound vain. But the desire that brings a woman to my office is rarely about vanity. It's about alignment—the yearning for her outer reflection to finally match who she knows herself to be inside.

Nashville Natural Notes–Practical wisdom from the consultation room

Confidence Should Look Like You

The goal of a Mommy Makeover is not to look like someone else.

It's to restore the natural shape your body once had—before pregnancy stretched and shifted things.

When results are balanced and proportional, they simply look like **the best version of you.**

One woman sat across from me, twisting her hands nervously. "I hate the way I look in jeans," she said. "I've tried everything—diet, exercise—but nothing fits right anymore." Another confessed, "I just want to get rid of this overhang. I feel like it's not even my body anymore." There's often shame in their voices, a hesitation to admit they've been quietly fighting themselves for years. But those words aren't about superficiality. They're about identity. They're the whispers of women ready to come home to themselves.

I remember one patient who was painfully shy during her first visit. She could barely meet my eyes during her preoperative photos. She kept apologizing for her appearance, for her decision, for even taking up space in the appointment. Two months after her surgery, she walked into the office transformed—not just physically, but emotionally. She laughed easily and said, "So when are you going to put my pictures on your website? I've already told five women to come see you." The same woman who had once hidden her reflection now wanted to celebrate it. That's not vanity—that's victory.

Plastic surgery is not a moral issue. It's a deeply personal one. The question isn't "Should I?" It's "Am I ready to see myself again?" *The transformation doesn't begin on the operating table. It begins in that quiet decision a woman makes—to give herself permission to matter again.*

For some, that decision takes years. For others, it happens in a single mirror glance that stops them cold. But every mom who chooses this path does it for one reason: she's tired of feeling disconnected from herself. And when she finally decides to bridge that gap, it's not selfish—it's healing.

Still, the term Mommy Makeover can sound confusing. What does it even mean? Many women assume it's one specific operation, a one-size-fits-all package. But that couldn't be further from the truth. A Mommy Makeover is not a single procedure—it's a personalized combination of surgeries or treatments designed to restore your body's harmony after childbirth. For one woman, it might mean tightening the abdomen and lifting the breasts. For another, it could include liposuction or labiaplasty to restore comfort and confidence. There's no fixed formula—only the balance that feels right for you.

When I meet with a patient, I don't start by talking about procedures. I start by asking questions—gentle, human questions that open a window into her story:

- What parts of your body do you love? Why?

- What areas cause you frustration or discomfort?
- How has your appearance changed since pregnancy?
- How would you like to feel when you look in the mirror?
- What would it mean for you to see that reflection again?

These questions aren't about perfection. They're about clarity. They help me understand not only her anatomy but her emotions—because both are vital to the outcome. The goal isn't to erase motherhood. It's to honor it and to rebuild strength, function, and confidence from it.

Every woman's journey is different. Some want to reclaim volume and lift in the breasts; others want to remove stretched-out skin around their core. Some are finally ready to address changes that have bothered them for years. And some simply want to feel whole again—to look in the mirror without flinching, to feel good slipping into clothes that reflect who they are, not who they used to be.

One mother once told me, "I feel guilty for even thinking about this. I should just be grateful." Gratitude and guilt often coexist in motherhood. You can love your children fiercely and still long for yourself. That's not contradiction—it's humanity. I've seen firsthand how a **mother's renewed confidence creates a ripple effect** that touches every corner of her life. Her laughter comes more easily. Her patience deepens. Her joy returns. And when she feels strong and radiant again, her family feels it too.

Of course, surgery isn't the right choice for everyone—and it's never a decision to rush. It requires mental, emotional, and physical readiness. It means preparing for change and embracing attention, both welcome and uninvited. It means knowing that some people will celebrate your courage while others may project their own insecurities onto your choice. The key is remembering that this decision belongs to you. It's your body, your story, and your restoration.

I remind every patient: you don't need anyone's permission but your own. And if you've carried a child, nourished a family, and given endlessly of yourself, you've already earned the right to feel beautiful again.

Yes, these surgeries require planning, investment, and time—but they are an investment in your well-being, not an indulgence. *A car depreciates, a house demands maintenance, but confidence compounds.* Imagine looking in the mirror every morning and feeling peace instead of frustration. That's not a luxury—it's a quiet revolution.

Still, a Mommy Makeover isn't magic. It won't fix what's broken in a relationship or erase every stress of motherhood. It can't make you twenty again. But it can remove the barriers that have kept you from seeing your reflection with kindness.

Every patient's journey begins and ends with one truth: You are not trying to change who you are. You are simply uncovering who's been there all along.

For many moms, that realization brings a mix of relief and unease. Relief because they finally see themselves again; unease because they've been conditioned to believe that caring for themselves must come at someone else's expense. The moment you give yourself permission to matter again, something else often surfaces—guilt. You may wonder if it's okay to want more, or whether loving your family fully means sacrificing every ounce of yourself. It's not selfish to refill your own tank. It's strength. It's stewardship.

In the next part of this journey, we'll talk about what happens after the decision—how to silence the guilt that whispers you shouldn't, how to protect your energy, and how to reconnect the body and mind that have carried you through so much.

For now, I want you to take a moment for reflection.

My Mommy Makeover is...

Write your own definition of a makeover—not one from an ad or a social feed, but your own. Start the sentence: "My mommy makeover is..." and finish it with a feeling, not a feature. Maybe it's "reclaiming my energy." Maybe it's "feeling comfortable in my skin." Maybe it's "seeing my reflection and smiling again." Whatever it is, write it down and hold it close—because the next step in your restoration isn't physical. It's learning to live freely in that permission you just gave yourself.

Because once you've given yourself permission to define your makeover, the next step is clarity—understanding where your body has been, where it is now, and what paths are available to you moving forward.

The Mommy Makeover Map

A simple guide to understanding the journey your body has taken—and the path forward from here.

Motherhood changes the body in powerful ways.

Some changes fade with time.

Others remain as lasting reminders of the incredible work your body performed.

This book is designed to guide you through those changes with clarity, compassion, and truth.

Think of the chapters ahead as a **map**—one that helps you understand:

• where your body has been
• where it is now
• what options exist if you want to restore parts of what pregnancy changed

Where Pregnancy Changes the Body

Pregnancy affects the body in several predictable areas.

Understanding these changes is the first step toward deciding what matters most to you.

The Breasts

Pregnancy and breastfeeding stretch breast tissue and supportive ligaments.

Common changes include:

• loss of fullness
• sagging (ptosis)
• enlarged areola
• asymmetry
• volume loss or gain

Chapters that explore solutions: **Chapters 17–21**

Procedures discussed:

• breast lift
• breast augmentation
• breast reduction
• lift with implants

Goal: **Restore balance and natural proportion.**

The Abdomen

The abdomen often experiences the most dramatic transformation.

Common changes include:

• overstretched skin
• striae- AKA stretch marks
• diastasis recti
(muscle separation)
• belly button distortion
• lower abdominal "apron"

Chapters that explore solutions:

Chapter 16 – The Tummy Truth

Procedures:

- tummy tuck
- mini tummy tuck
- extended tummy tuck
- belt lipectomy

Goal: **Restore strength and stability to your center.**

The Waist and Flanks

Even after weight loss, some fat deposits remain resistant to diet and exercise.

Commonly called:

- love handles
- muffin top
- flank fullness

Chapters that explore solutions:

Chapter 14 & 15 – Fat distribution and Liposuction

Goal: **Reveal the natural curves of your waistline.**

The Intimate Area

Childbirth can also affect vaginal and labial tissues.

Concerns may include:

- discomfort
- stretching
- reduced sexual confidence

Chapter that explores solutions:

Chapter 22 — The Intimate Restoration

Possible options:

- labiaplasty
- vaginal rejuvenation

Goal: **Restore comfort, confidence, and self-respect.**

The Four Pillars of a Mommy Makeover

A Mommy Makeover is not one single surgery.

It is a **customized combination of procedures** designed to restore the areas most affected by pregnancy.

Most plans fall into four major categories.

1. Breast Restoration

Restoring the shape, volume, or comfort of the breasts.

Procedures may include:

- breast lift
- breast augmentation
- breast lift with augmentation
- breast reduction

Goal: **Restore proportion and femininity.**

Chapters: **17–21**

2. Core Restoration

Repairing abdominal muscles and removing excess skin.

Procedures may include:

- tummy tuck
- extended tummy tuck
- belt lipectomy

Goal: **Restore strength and stability to the body's center.**

Chapter: **16**

3. Contour Refinement

Removing stubborn fat deposits that remain despite healthy lifestyle habits.

Procedures may include:

- liposuction of the waist
- flank contouring
- lower back contouring

Goal: **Restore the silhouette beneath the skin.**

Chapter: **14 & 15**

4. Feminine Confidence

Addressing intimate anatomical changes after childbirth.

Procedures may include:

- labiaplasty
- vaginal rejuvenation

Goal: **Restore comfort, confidence, and intimacy.**

Chapter: **22**

The Journey Through This Book

Each section of this book guides you through a different stage of transformation.

Think of it as moving step-by-step along the map.

PART I — Seeing Yourself Again

Chapters 1–5 explore the emotional reality many moms experience after pregnancy.

Topics include:

- body identity
- guilt vs self-care
- the myth of "bouncing back"

Goal: **Replace shame with understanding.**

PART II — Preparing for Your Comeback

Chapters 6–13 help you prepare mentally and practically for change.

Topics include:

- making the decision
- choosing a surgeon
- emotional preparation
- recovery expectations

Goal: **Move from guilt to agency.**

PART III — Rebuilding Beautiful

Chapters 14–22 explore the tools of transformation.

Topics include:

- liposuction
- tummy tuck surgery
- breast procedures
- labiaplasty

Goal: **Empower you with knowledge and options.**

PART IV — The Confidence Afterglow

Chapters 23–24 explore what happens after transformation.

Topics include:

- identity
- confidence
- family ripple effects
- long-term wellbeing

Goal: **Help you live fully in your restored reflection.**

Final Thought of the Mommy Makeover Map

Pregnancy changed your body because it carried life.

Understanding those changes is not about criticizing the past.

It's about making informed, compassionate choices for the future.

And wherever you are on this journey—**you are allowed to feel strong, confident, and at home in your body again.**

The Mommy Makeover Confidence Pyramid

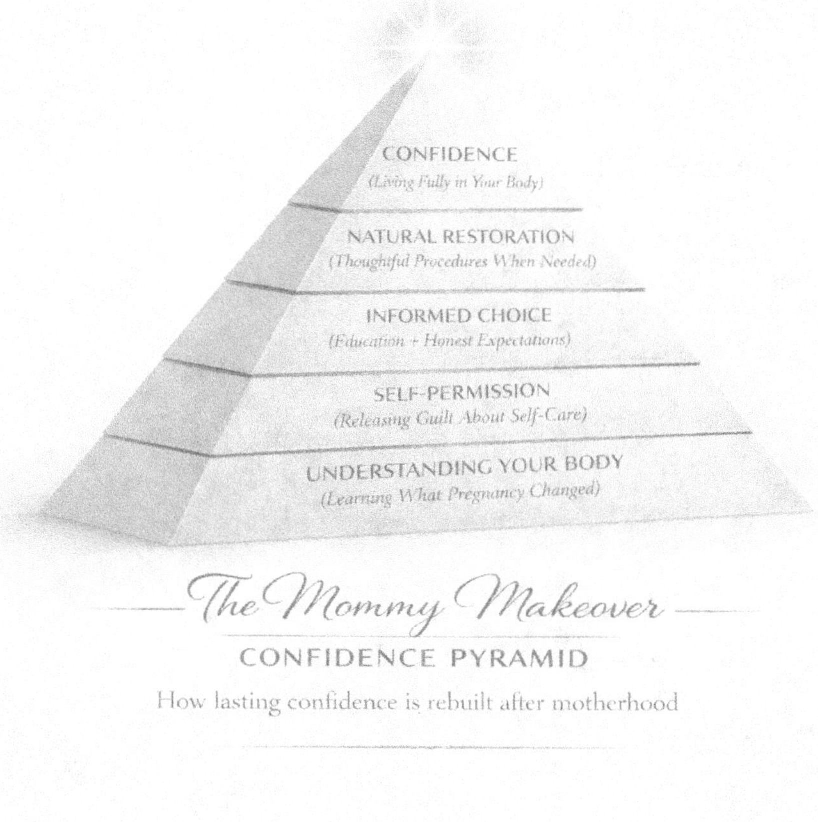
CONFIDENCE
(Living Fully in Your Body)
NATURAL RESTORATION
(Thoughtful Procedures When Needed)
INFORMED CHOICE
(Education + Honest Expectations)
SELF-PERMISSION
(Releasing Guilt About Self-Care)
UNDERSTANDING YOUR BODY
(Learning What Pregnancy Changed)
The Mommy Makeover
CONFIDENCE PYRAMID
How lasting confidence is rebuilt after motherhood

Layer 1 — Understanding Your Body

The foundation

Confidence begins with knowledge.

Many women blame themselves for changes that are actually biological results of pregnancy.

Understanding the anatomy of what changed—and why—removes unnecessary guilt.

When women learn about:

- abdominal muscle separation
- stretched skin
- breast tissue changes
- hormonal fat redistribution

they often experience something powerful... relief

Relevant chapters:

- The Myths of the Bounce Back
- The Post-Baby Body Reality Check
- The Tummy Truth
- The Breast Story

Layer 2 — Self-Permission

Releasing guilt

For many mothers, the hardest step is giving themselves permission to focus on their own wellbeing.

Women often ask:

"Is it selfish to want my body back?"

The truth is that caring for yourself does not diminish your love for your family.

In fact, when a mom feels confident and energized, the entire household benefits.

Relevant chapters:

- When Love and Guilt Collide
- The Body-Mind Connection
- The Moment You Decide You're Worth It

Layer 3 — Informed Choice

Learning your options

Once guilt fades, curiosity begins.

This stage involves learning what is actually possible and what is realistic.

That includes understanding:

- liposuction
- tummy tuck surgery
- breast procedures

- intimate rejuvenation
- recovery expectations

Knowledge creates empowered decisions.

Relevant chapters:

- Preparing for Your Comeback
- Choosing the Right Surgeon

Layer 4 — Natural Restoration

Thoughtful transformation

When surgery is chosen thoughtfully, the goal is always **balance and proportion**, not dramatic change.

The best aesthetic results look natural.

Friends may not know exactly what changed.

They simply notice that you look healthy, vibrant, and comfortable in your own skin.

Relevant chapters:

- Liposuction
- The Tummy Truth
- Breast Procedures
- Labiaplasty and the Art of Intimate Restoration.

Layer 5 — Confidence

The real transformation

The final transformation isn't visible on an operating table.

It's confidence that shows up in everyday life.

Women often describe:

- standing taller
- enjoying photos again
- feeling comfortable in clothes
- reconnecting with their partners

Confidence ripples outward into family life, relationships, and daily energy.

Relevant chapters:

- Becoming Visible Again
- The Ripple Effect

Mommy Makeover Readiness Quiz

A quick check-in with your body, your confidence, and your goals.

Motherhood asks extraordinary things of a woman's body.

Some women feel completely at peace with the changes that follow.

Others quietly wonder whether they could feel more comfortable, confident, or connected to themselves again.

This short quiz is not about telling you whether you *should* pursue a Mommy Makeover.

It simply helps you reflect on whether **the idea is worth exploring further.**

Answer honestly.

Scoring Your Answers

For each question in the **Mommy Makeover Readiness Quiz**, assign:

- **2 points** — Strong yes / resonates strongly
- **1 point** — Somewhat / occasionally true
- **0 points** — Not really true for me

Total your score.

Maximum score: **30 points**

Part 1 — The "Me Time" Question

1. Do you ever catch yourself wondering, "When is it my turn?"

- 2=daily,
- 1=frequently,
- 0=What even is that?

2. Have you sacrificed a lot—or almost everything—for your family's needs?

- 2= Strong Yes.
- 1=Somewhat.
- 0= Not really true for me.

3. Do you sometimes feel like you lost a part of yourself while caring for your children?

- 2= Strong Yes, I don't recognize myself anymore.
- 1=Somewhat, I just don't feel like myself anymore.
- 0= Not really true for me, that's part of being a Mom.

4. When you imagine doing something purely for yourself, do you feel excitement?

- 2 = Yes
- 1 = Unsure
- 0 = You feel guilt

5. Do you believe plastic surgery will solve your personal or relationship problems?

- 2= No way – a Mommy Makeover is purely a cosmetic treat for me.
- 1= I don't expect plastic surgery to solve my problems, but I need a Mommy Makeover for my own sanity and wellbeing.
- 0= Are you kidding me?! If my boobs were perkier/butt was tighter/tummy was slimmer, most of my problems would be solved.

Part 2 — How You Feel in Your Body Questions

6. How much time do you devote to your own health and fitness?

- 2=I manage to hit the gym several days a week, but my tummy just won't tighten!
- 1= Not much - I give everything I have to my kids and have no time for myself.
- 0=Zero. Health and fitness were never really my strong suit, even before kids.

7. When is the last time you wore a bikini confidently in public?

- 2= Since before my babies were born – but I used to rock one every summer!
- 1= Too long ago to remember. Besides, who has time to go to the beach or pool?
- 0= Never – I've always been too overweight and out of shape.

8. What part(s) of your post-baby body bothers you the most?

- 2= I don't recognize my breasts, body, labia anymore, and it's only gotten worse since having children.
- 1= Mainly my breasts – they've never been the same since I stopped breastfeeding.
- 0= I still have floppy skin and stretch marks on my belly!

9. Do you often use food terms like "muffin top" or "flapjacks" to describe your body parts?

- 2= I complain about my muffin top so often, I've actually made myself hungry a time or two!
- 1= Definitely not...but I do refer to my "saddle bags."
- 0= I try not to disparage myself (even if I secretly think my breasts resemble my kids' breakfast).

10. Since having children, has poor body image stopped you from participating in activities?

- 2= I never let my "mom bod" hold me back – it could just use a little boost, that's all.
- 1= I've always been self-conscious about my body, so I've often passed up swimming, dancing, playing sports – you name it
- 0= I had to give my bikini a burial at sea! No more two-pieces for this mama.

Part 3 — Practical Readiness Questions

11. Have you given your body enough time after pregnancy to

recover naturally? (I recommend waiting at least 6-12 months after childbirth)

- 2= 6-12 Months
- 1= 3-6 Months
- 0= I just got home from the hospital

12. Are you planning to have more children?

- 2= Nope. Put a fork in me, I'm done!
- 1= I'm done for now...but you never know.
- 0= Another pregnancy is definitely in my future

13. Have you discussed getting a Mommy Makeover with your partner, children and/or friends and family?

- 2= Yes, and we're all on the same page – including on my Vision Board.
- 1= No, I actually hadn't considered a Mommy Makeover as a real possibility until this moment.
- 0= I've brought up weight-loss surgery to my partner in the past – does that count?

14. Can you arrange for the help and recovery time required after a Mommy Makeover?

- 2= Done and done! I already have a recovery plan in place.
- 1= If I could handle childbirth, then caring for a newborn, I'm sure I can handle a little cosmetic surgery. I got this!

- 0= I'll have to think this through, but I should be able to prepare with enough notice.

15. What is your number one motivation for considering plastic surgery?

- 2= I am ready to reclaim my Confidence, Connection and my Reflection
- 1= I'm frustrated with working hard to get my pre-baby body back with little results.
- 0= My body just hasn't been the same since baby and I feel like surgery would boost my self-esteem and give me a fresh start.

What Your Answers Might Mean

If several questions resonated with you, it may simply mean this:

You're not alone.

Many women reach a point after pregnancy where they want to reconnect with their bodies—not out of vanity, but out of a desire to feel **comfortable, confident, and whole again.**

Exploring your options doesn't mean you're rejecting motherhood.

It means you're acknowledging that **the woman who carried life deserves care too.**

One Final Question

Before moving forward, answer this honestly:

If I could feel strong, comfortable, and confident in my body again...
how would that change my life?

Write your answer here:

____

____

____

Interpret Your Score

0–9 points *Almost Fit for a Mommy Makeover – With a little prep work, a Mommy Makeover could be in your future!*

You currently may be in the Curiosity Stage

You may simply be becoming aware of the changes pregnancy made to your body.

At this stage most women are:

- noticing changes
- learning what is normal
- exploring their options

What to read next:
Chapters 1–5 (Seeing Yourself Again)

Goal:
Replace confusion with understanding.

10–19 points *Mommy Makeover Material – You are a great candidate for a Mommy Makeover!*

You're likely in the Research Stage

You've likely spent some time thinking about your body changes and what might help.

Women in this stage are often:

- researching procedures
- asking friends for experiences
- learning what surgery actually involves

What to read next:
Chapters 6–13 (Preparing for Your Comeback)

Goal:
Move from curiosity to informed decision-making.

20–30 points *MORE than Mommy Makeover Ready – You're an ideal candidate for a Mommy Makeover! What are you waiting for?*

You are in the "Ready to Consult" Stage

You may be ready to speak with a surgeon and explore your options seriously.

Women in this stage often:

- have tried exercise and lifestyle changes first
- understand what bothers them most
- feel emotionally ready to consider change

What to read next:

Chapters 14–22 (Rebuilding Beautiful)

Goal:

Understand procedures and what transformation realistically looks like.

Gentle Reminder

Your score is **not a prescription**.

It simply reflects where you might be in your personal journey.

Every woman moves through these stages differently.

I invite you to continue reading to develop familiarity with the Mommy Makeover concept/procedures and decide if this is a journey you want to take to reclaim your confidence, connection and reflection.

The 10 Truths Every Mom Deserves to Hear

Motherhood asks extraordinary things of a woman's body.

Some of those changes fade with time.
Some do not.

Before we go any further, there are a few truths every mom deserves to hear.

1. Your body did not fail you.

It stretched.
It adapted.
It carried life.

That is not failure.

That is biology doing something extraordinary.

2. "Bouncing back" is a myth.

Pregnancy changes muscles, skin, and connective tissue in ways diet and exercise alone cannot always reverse.

That doesn't mean you did something wrong.

It means your body did something powerful.

3. Wanting to feel comfortable in your body is not vanity.

Confidence is not selfish.

When a woman feels strong and at home in her body again, it changes how she moves through the world.

4. You are allowed to take care of yourself.

For many moms, caring for everyone else becomes the default.

But restoring yourself is not taking away from your family.

It often gives more of you back to them.

5. You are not the only one who feels this way.

Thousands of women quietly experience the same thoughts:

"Is this really my body now?"

You are not alone in asking that question.

6. Your worth is not measured by your waistline.

Your value was never determined by stretch marks, loose skin, or breast shape.

Your worth was already established the moment you became a mother—and long before that.

7. Transformation is not about perfection.

The goal is not a flawless body.

The goal is alignment between how you feel inside and how you show up in the world.

8. Surgery is a tool, not the definition of beauty.

For some women, procedures restore comfort and confidence.

For others, understanding their bodies is enough.

Both paths are valid.

9. Confidence creates a ripple effect.

When a mom feels strong and visible again, it affects everything:

Her posture.
Her energy.
Her relationships.
Her children.

Confidence is contagious.

10. You are allowed to become yourself again.

Motherhood transforms a woman.

But it doesn't erase who she is.

Sometimes the most powerful moment in a mom's journey is simply realizing:

She is allowed to step fully into the woman she has become.

Closing Reflection

Your body carried life.

If part of your journey now includes restoring parts of what pregnancy changed, that decision is not about erasing motherhood.

It is about honoring the woman who lived it.

CHAPTER 4

When Love and Guilt Collide

You give yourself to everyone else—until there's nothing left for you.

This isn't a flaw. It's love. It's instinct. It's what makes you *you.* It's what makes you "mom". But somewhere between preschool drop-off, bedtime stories, and endless loads of laundry, something sacred often slips away—the space inside you that once belonged to *you alone.*

5:30 a.m. The baby stirs. You're already half-awake, anticipating it. You warm a bottle quietly, hoping not to wake the others. Too late. Here come the boys.

6:00 a.m. Breakfast. One wants cereal, one wants eggs, one isn't hungry. Backpacks, lunch boxes, chaos. You catch a glimpse of yourself in the microwave reflection and wonder when you last sat down to eat a meal that wasn't half a leftover sandwich.

7:45 a.m. The house finally exhales. You tell yourself you'll rest after the baby goes down. But guilt overrides. There's laundry, dishes, a floor to sweep, a pantry to organize. Makeup? Maybe in the car. Breakfast? Maybe tomorrow.

You start each day hopeful and think you'll be fine. Most times your thoughts revolve around your kids. You worry. Are you teaching them well, are they making the right friends, fitting in, have we signed up for the right activities, will they grow up to be kind, thoughtful, and empathetic, etc.? You make it through the day, barely, and still don't exercise or even get a short nap.

And somehow, this rhythm repeats—day after day, love after love, until you realize you've given everything you have... except permission to stop.

Most mothers don't consciously choose to put themselves last. It happens gradually, in a thousand small acts of love. They are just so focused on everyone else in the family, they just never get around to attending to themselves, they sort of get "forgotten" in the shuffle. But the truth is, uninterrupted giving has a cost. Psychologists call it *empathy fatigue*—the slow, invisible burnout that happens when your compassion reserves are continually spent without being replenished.

When you give endlessly without receiving rest, acknowledgment, or care, your body interprets it as depletion. Cortisol levels rise. Sleep patterns shift. Joy flattens. And before long, you start confusing exhaustion for normalcy. That's why self-care isn't indulgence—it's biology. The nervous system can only give so much before it demands balance.

I've watched it in my own home. My mother, and later my wife, have each given endlessly—through pregnancy, breastfeeding, sleepless nights, football carpools, piano lessons. My wife likes to remind me that something 'breaks' with each pregnancy. And she's right. As the baby grows, for instance, the fibrous band of tissue that runs down the middle of the abdomen can become permanently stretched out of shape.

Many women end up with what my patients call a 'dunlap'—a Southern term that was new to this New Jersey native. It means muffin top, pooch, or love handles when referring to the abdomen, as in 'My belly has done lapped over my belt.' That one always makes me smile—but it's also a reminder that these changes, while universal, are not trivial. They're physical records of motherhood's devotion. The love they give is beautiful. But the toll it takes is real. Every mom I meet has made that same trade: self for service, joy for duty, body for family. But here's the truth most mothers never hear—you're allowed to give to yourself too.

One of my patients, Kristin, came to see me in her early thirties. The mother of two, she was healthy and active but discouraged by the changes two pregnancies had left behind. Her breasts were deflated; her stomach carried an overhang no amount of crunches could flatten. She loved her kids, but she missed feeling confident in her own skin.

She worried her husband might disapprove when she brought up surgery. To her surprise, he didn't hesitate. 'If this will make you feel better,' he said, 'then I'm all for it.' That was all Kristin needed to make the call. Her Mommy Makeover included a breast lift with conservative augmentation and a tummy tuck. When I saw her at her follow-up, she looked radiant. Her smile was easy. Her confidence filled the room. She told me she went to the neighborhood pool without hesitation for the first time in years. She laughed and said, 'I finally feel like me again.' And her whole family felt that lightness, too.

This is what I mean when I say self-care is strength. Kristin didn't do it to impress anyone else. She did it because she'd reached the point where her reflection no longer matched her spirit. That dissonance isn't vanity—it's a sign that something inside needs restoration.

The question I ask my patients isn't, 'Are you ready for surgery?' It's, 'Are you ready to see yourself as worthy of the same care you give everyone else?' Taking time, spending money, or scheduling recovery doesn't make you selfish. It makes you sustainable.

You need the proverbial oxygen mask. If you collapse from depletion, the entire ecosystem of your family feels it.

Every mother knows the physical sacrifices of pregnancy and childbirth—the swelling, stretching, sleeplessness, and hormones. But few realize how much of that sacrifice lingers quietly, reshaping not just their bodies but their minds. Even after the sleepless nights fade, many moms carry the invisible residue of self-denial. That's where guilt hides. It whispers, 'You should be grateful. You shouldn't want more.'

Gratitude and guilt often live side by side in motherhood. You can love your children fiercely and still miss the woman you were before them. You can be grateful for the gift of life and still grieve the cost of it. The truth is, those feelings don't cancel each other out—they coexist. And learning to hold both is where healing begins.

So when is it time? When is it Mommy time?

Some of my patients have waited years, even decades, to make themselves a priority. Others come in as soon as their bodies have healed and their hearts are ready. There's no perfect moment—only readiness. **Readiness looks like exhaustion giving way to resolve**. Like a whisper that says, 'I've done everything for them. Maybe it's time to do something for me.'

A Mommy Makeover has the best results when a mother has done what she can to restore herself naturally—through nutrition, gentle movement, and patience. Then, when her body has plateaued and her spirit still yearns for more, that's when we can help. The better shape you're in—physically and emotionally—the better you'll heal. But if you're waiting for a perfect time, it will never come. Kids will still need rides. Laundry will still pile up. Life doesn't pause. You have to choose to step into it. You have to choose you for once.

This reminds me of my patient Mandy, who used to bring her teenage daughter in with her for her post operative visits, to teach her that caring for yourself as a mother is actually a healthy act of love. Here's how she explained it to her 13-year-old: "As a mom, I sacrificed to have children. My body has changed, and some of those changes I can't undo. What I've given to you I wouldn't trade for the world, but now I'm doing something for myself." I think that's a positive and very healthy approach.

That choice isn't indulgence. It's a declaration. It says: 'I'm still here, and I'm worth caring for.' And when you do, the ripple effect begins. Your family sees it. Your children see it. Your partner sees it. And they all benefit from a mother who feels whole.

The Oxygen Mask Test

Tonight, take a breath and try what I call *The Oxygen Mask Test.*

Ask yourself one simple question:

What three daily acts refill my tank?

It might be a walk without your phone. Ten quiet minutes of reading. Eating breakfast while it's still warm. Write them down. Then make them non-negotiable—small rituals that remind you *your needs* matter.

Because caring for yourself doesn't mean loving your family less. It means showing them what real love looks like—love that sustains, not depletes.

And when you begin to refill your own tank, you'll feel something unexpected: your body exhaling. Because your body remembers everything—the giving, the fatigue, the moments of holding your breath.

In the next chapter, we'll explore how your body carries those memories—and how to release them with compassion.

CHAPTER 5
The Body–Mind Connection

Your body remembers everything—birth, stress, and even silence. It remembers the late nights you spent pacing with a feverish baby. The tension you held in your shoulders while holding your breath through a tantrum. The way you curled/ folded into yourself when you didn't feel beautiful. The body never forgets. It carries the stories your words never said out loud.

In my years as a plastic surgeon, I've learned that every scar, every stretch mark, every curve tells a story far deeper than anatomy. When I examine a patient, I'm not just looking at skin or muscle. I'm listening—to the history written beneath the surface. To the fatigue she hides behind her smile. To the grief she's tucked neatly under her Spanx. To the way her body has quietly absorbed the weight of motherhood, marriage, and the relentless expectation to 'hold it all together.'

After childbirth, the body transforms in ways that are both miraculous and, at times, devastatingly humbling. But what many women don't realize is that these physical changes are often intertwined with emotional ones. The muscles that stretched to carry life can hold the tension of that responsibility for years. The breath that once expanded with anticipation can become shallow with stress. The heart that grew with love can also carry the ache of disconnection—from self, from partner, from peace.

I've had women tell me, 'I feel heavy, even though I'm back to my pre-pregnancy weight.' Others say, 'I can't seem to stand up straight anymore,' or 'I'm always tired, even when I sleep.' These are not just physical complaints—they're the echoes of emotional strain that the body has translated into posture, breath, and fatigue.

There's a reason for this. The nervous system doesn't separate physical and emotional stress. When your body perceives threat—whether it's lack of sleep, a crying baby, or self-criticism—it reacts the same way. Adrenaline spikes. Cortisol floods. Muscles tighten. The fight-or-flight response becomes your new normal. Over time, this chronic activation exhausts the body and fogs the mind. You start to forget what relaxation even feels like.

Healing, then, isn't just about surgery, exercise, or diet—it's about *awareness.* It's about learning to listen to what your body is trying to tell you, to respond with compassion instead of correction. In my practice, I often tell patients, 'Your recovery starts the moment you decide to treat your body like an ally instead of an enemy.'

That begins with simple awareness. Pay attention to how your body feels when you walk into a room, when you look in the mirror, when you catch your reflection by accident. Notice if you tighten, shrink, sigh, or smile. These are clues—your body's way of speaking.

One of my patients, Emily, taught me this lesson early in my career. She came in for a tummy tuck after two pregnancies and a decade of 'doing everything right'—eating well, exercising, working, parenting, giving. Her results were beautiful, but six months later she still felt disconnected. She said, 'My body looks healed, but I still feel broken.'

I encouraged her to start paying attention not to how her body looked, but to how it *felt.* When she returned three months later, she said something I'll never forget: 'I realized I've been holding my stomach in for ten years.' It wasn't vanity—it was vigilance. Her core muscles had been braced against stress for so long that relaxation felt foreign. The moment she exhaled and released that tension, she said she cried—not from sadness, but from relief.

That's what I mean when I say the body remembers. Sometimes it remembers trauma; sometimes it remembers protection. Either way, part of healing is teaching your body that it's safe again—to soften, to trust, to expand.

From a medical perspective, this is called *somatic awareness*—the conscious attention to physical sensations as a pathway to emotional well-being. When you start noticing how your body responds to emotion—tight chest with anxiety, shallow breath with guilt, slumped posture with shame—you gain the power to interrupt the cycle. Instead of pushing through discomfort, you can pause and ask, 'What is my body trying to tell me right now?'

Self-compassion is the medicine that allows this awareness to work. When you treat yourself with kindness, your body feels it. The 'Fight or Flight' mode-- the sympathetic nervous system-- can relax. The parasympathetic nervous system—your 'rest and restore' mode—activates and takes over. Your muscles soften. Your breathing deepens. Your digestion improves. Your blood flow improves. Healing accelerates. This is not abstract—it's physiology.

So much of modern motherhood demands suppression. Hold it in. Hold it together. Hold everyone else up. But the truth is, healing happens when you start letting go—of tension, of guilt, of the unrealistic expectations you've carried. When you start releasing what's been held too tightly, you create space for peace to return.

I often tell my patients: **surgery can restore the canvas, but only you can restore the connection**. The way you inhabit your body after healing determines how long your results will last—not just physically, but emotionally. If you continue to carry shame or resentment, your posture, your breath, even your energy will bear that weight. But if you approach your body with gratitude, it will respond like any relationship—it will soften, open, and thrive. And heal quicker too. As your surgeon, I am deeply concerned with your physical healing, yes, but I am all about the 'whole mom' being healthy. Those transformations are the most magical ones.

Body Gratitude Meditation

So how do you begin? You start small. You start with acknowledgment. Before you go to bed tonight, place a hand on your heart and another on your abdomen. Breathe in deeply, feeling your chest and belly rise. Then exhale slowly. Whisper a quiet thank-you—to the body that carried your children, to the heart that kept loving even when it was tired, to the mind that kept going when it wanted to quit.

This is your body gratitude meditation. It takes two minutes, but its effects are profound.

Close your eyes and name three things your body has carried you through—birth, loss, joy, recovery. Say them out loud. Let the words land. Then, with your next breath, say: 'You did it. Thank you.'

That is where healing begins—not in striving, but in stillness. Not in judgment, but in grace.

Your body remembers everything. But starting today, it can also remember your kindness.

In the next chapter, we'll explore what it means to move forward from that awareness—to align your physical recovery with your emotional growth, and to write a new story for both.

PART II
PREPARING FOR YOUR COMEBACK

From guilt to growth: reclaiming agency over your transformation.

CHAPTER 6

The Moment You Decide You're Worth It

The hardest part isn't the surgery—it's giving yourself permission.

In every consultation I've ever had, there's a moment that comes before the decision. It's not when we discuss incisions, anesthesia, or recovery. It's quieter than that. It's the pause, the deep breath, the hesitant question: 'Do you think I'm being selfish?' And my answer is always the same: No. You're being honest.

For so many women, the hardest battle isn't physical—it's emotional. It's not about whether they want to look better; it's whether they feel they're *allowed* to. They stand at the intersection of longing and guilt, looking both ways, afraid to step forward. They've spent years giving—to children, partners, parents, communities—and they've learned to equate selflessness with worth. But when everything you give flows outward, eventually, something inside you runs dry.

This chapter is about that moment—the moment you decide you're worth it.

I see many mothers who feel guilty even considering doing the littlest things for themselves, let alone plastic surgery. It seems to stem from the inherent nature of moms to think of everyone else first and always put themselves last. Let me ask you: If all the logistics of childcare and household duties were met, all your questions answered, and all your concerns addressed, would you then give yourself permission to have plastic surgery? Do you feel you're worth it? Only you can answer that question. But I'll tell you this: if you are a mom who has sacrificed to carry a baby, gone through childbirth, and continued that sacrifice every single day since, you've already earned the right to give to yourself.

I've seen entire families blossom from having a mother who feels confident in her own skin. This kind of transformation doesn't just affect one person—it ripples outward. This is the "**ripple effect of plastic surgery**" that I've talked about before. And it's AWESOME. When a mom stands taller, smiles wider, and feels proud again, everyone around her benefits. The energy in the home shifts. Children notice it. Spouses notice it. The world notices it. That's what confidence does—it quietly restores balance.

Still, I understand the hesitation. You want to be responsible. You worry about timing, safety, finances. You tell yourself, 'Maybe next year.' But readiness isn't about perfection—it's about peace. Here's how I help my patients discern whether they're truly ready.

The Readiness Markers

****Emotional**:** You're no longer making the decision from a place of desperation or self-criticism, but from love. You're doing this *for* yourself, not *against* yourself.

****Relational**:** You've had an honest conversation with your support system—your partner, family, or closest friend—and you feel understood, not judged.

Financial: You've evaluated your investment with clarity, not guilt. You see this as a long-term investment in your quality of life, not a one-time indulgence.

Spiritual: You feel a quiet peace in your decision—a sense that this step aligns with who you are becoming, not who you're trying to impress.

When these four areas begin to align, the question shifts from *Can I?* to *Why not me?*

And that's when you know you're ready.

Readiness doesn't end with peace of mind—it extends into preparation. In my practice, I teach every patient to make sure she has *four yeses* before proceeding:

The Right Patient: Are you physically healthy, emotionally stable, and choosing this for *you*—not for anyone else?

The Right Surgeon: Is your surgeon board-certified, experienced, and someone you trust with not just your safety, but your story?

The Right Procedure(s): Have you identified the procedures that align with your goals and anatomy—not what social media says you 'should' do?

The Right Timing: Have you allowed your body enough time to recover from pregnancy, finished breastfeeding, and coordinated support for your recovery?

When you can confidently answer *yes* to all four, you've laid the foundation for not only a safe surgery, but a meaningful transformation. We'll explore each of these in greater detail later in the book—but for now, let's turn to one of the most important: *safety.*

Safety First—Is a Mommy Makeover Safe?

The usual procedures for a Mommy Makeover are very safe. If you have a skilled, board-certified plastic surgeon working in a modern, accredited operating room, complications are rare. From my experience, most moms are relatively young and healthy without serious medical problems. And that includes today's generation of moms in their 30s and 40s—ages that used to sound 'late' for motherhood, but now represent strength, stability, and wisdom.

The thinking today is that 60 is the new 40—and 40 is really young. Those factors make the surgery and healing process much easier. Healthy moms can safely undergo several procedures at once and recover beautifully. We even joke in the office, 'Why waste a good general anesthesia on only one surgery?' When performed together, procedures share a single anesthetic, one recovery period, and one block of downtime. The overall discomfort isn't much greater, but the benefits are multiplied.

Advantages of combining procedures include:

- A single anesthesia session (potentially safer)
- A single recovery period
- Similar pain levels to single surgeries
- Household and childcare arrangements made only once
- Potential cost savings on facility and anesthesia fees

Of course, not every patient is a candidate for combination surgery. If you have health concerns—such as severe hypertension, uncontrolled diabetes, or are an active smoker—your surgeon may advise postponing surgery. I ask all my patients who smoke to quit at least six weeks before surgery and remain smoke-free until fully healed (about 3 months later). Smoking restricts blood flow and slows recovery, but with preparation and guidance, most women achieve outstanding outcomes.

The most common pre-surgical challenge I see isn't physical—it's emotional. Many moms arrive in my office feeling low, tired, even mildly depressed from years of self-neglect. And yet, when they finally take this step, the transformation is more than cosmetic. I've seen a Mommy Makeover lift not only bodies but spirits. When a woman reclaims her reflection, she often reclaims her joy.

There's a specific moment during consultations that always gives me goosebumps.

It happens when I realize she's "there. "She's given herself permission.

Even in her shyness or vulnerability—standing in the exam room, nervous about the physical evaluation—I can often see the result before we ever begin. Not just the physical transformation, but the emotional one.

As I examine, I talk her through every step. I'll gently pinch the skin at her waist, measure her breasts, or trace along her abdomen, showing her in the mirror exactly what can be removed, repositioned, uncovered. I might say, "This is where we'll restore your waistline," or, "Here's where your nipple will sit again." And then I'll grab that small fold above her C-section scar and smile, "We can get rid of this."

Sometimes, I see the moment she believes me. Her eyes widen. Her posture lifts. It's as if she walks through the mirror and meets her future self—the one who's already healed, already confident, already home in her skin.

That's the moment the surgery truly begins—not in the operating room, but in her mind. When she can finally visualize the result with me, she steps into the transformation fully, not as a patient, but as a partner in her own renewal.

And for me, it never gets old. Every time, it's awesome.

Paying for Your Mommy Makeover—You're Worth It

This is where many women pause. They can justify any expense for their children—the sports camp, the braces, the dance recital—but struggle when it comes to spending on themselves. It's a cultural script that's hard to unlearn: the good mom sacrifices everything. But what if true generosity starts with wholeness? What if caring for yourself *is* a gift to your family?

A Mommy Makeover is not an indulgence. It's an investment—a one-time restoration that pays dividends in confidence and well-being for years to come. You see confidence compounds. Unlike a car, it doesn't depreciate; unlike a house, it doesn't require endless maintenance. It's a decision that changes how you move through the world, how you meet your own eyes in the mirror.

I often tell my patients: try to stop thinking about the price and start thinking about the value. How many times a day do you look in the mirror and feel that pang—'I wish I could fix this'? Now imagine looking every day and feeling peace instead of frustration. Would that be worth a penny each time? A dime? If so, you've already covered the investment many times over.

Our team helps every patient plan responsibly. Some pay upfront. Others choose financing or installment options. There's no shame in either path. The key is not whether you can afford it immediately—but whether you can afford to keep waiting to feel like yourself again.

Linda, a mom who struggled to find her worthiness in this decision, delayed for years. Finally, she took the plunge and completed her Mommy Makeover. During one of her post-operative visits, she was just so excited about her results and her decision to honor herself with this. "It's probably the best," she trailed off..."Well, I got married, I had kids so... **one of the best decisions** I've made in my life." As a third place winner, I'll take that behind husband and kids any day. 😉

The Readiness Reflection

Take a quiet moment today and ask yourself: *What's really stopping me?* Is it time, money, fear, or something deeper? Write down each hesitation on a piece of paper. Then next to it, ask: *Is this truth, or is it fear?* You may find that most of what's holding you back isn't reality—it's conditioning.

When you look at that list, ask yourself one more question: *If I remove guilt from the equation, what would I choose?*

That question alone has changed countless women's lives.

The Permission Slip

This final step is simple but powerful. We all know about the permission slips required at school for our kids various activities...field trips, doctor appointments, early pickups from school. This one, however, is for you. Take a blank sheet of paper and write at the top:

Permission Slip

Today, I give myself permission to do something that brings me peace, confidence, and joy.

Sign your name beneath it. Date it. Fold it up and keep it somewhere close—a drawer, your nightstand, your wallet. You don't need anyone else's signature but your own.

Because the truth is, readiness doesn't start in the body. It starts in the mind. And the moment you give yourself permission, you've already begun to heal.

In the next chapter, we'll talk about what happens when that decision turns into action—how preparation, partnership, and perspective make all the difference in your journey.

CHAPTER 7

Conversations That Change Everything

"You're not asking for approval—you're inviting understanding."

Every transformation starts as a private decision, but sooner or later, it becomes a conversation. A Mommy Makeover is not just about the body—it's about connection. And when that connection involves spouses, children, friends, or family, the way you communicate your 'why' can change everything.

I've seen countless women struggle with what to say, or whether to say anything at all. They imagine their partner's disapproval or a friend's judgment before ever speaking the words aloud. By the time they sit in my consultation room, they've already had five imaginary arguments in their head. I gently tell them, 'Let's not have the whole fight before you've even had the conversation.'

The truth is, most of the time, people who love you just want to understand you. They want to know you're safe. They want to know your happiness isn't coming at a cost to your well-being. And they want to see you light up when you talk about how this choice will make you feel. When you lead with honesty and confidence, you don't need anyone's permission—you're simply inviting understanding.

--Talking With Your Spouse or Partner

Discussing a Mommy Makeover with your partner can feel daunting. Sometimes, it's not about money at all—it's about vulnerability. To bring up surgery means admitting there are parts of yourself you wish to change. And for many women, that can feel like confessing failure. You can juggle a household, a career, and a family—but you can't seem to fix your body, and that can sting.

As a doctor, I can assure you: the "perfect supermom" doesn't exist. And as a husband, I can tell you—sometimes men just don't know what to say. When you finally bring up the topic, the most common response I hear about is, 'But you look beautiful to me just the way you are.' It's said with love—but it can feel dismissive when you've spent years quietly aching to feel like yourself again.

So how do you talk about it? You start by being honest and compassionate—with him and with yourself.

Tell him what this means to you—not what's wrong, but what you hope to reclaim. Say something like, 'I love that you see me as beautiful. I just want to feel that way too.' This opens a door to connection instead of confrontation.

Most partners aren't resistant because of vanity or ego—they're afraid. Men are wired to protect. It's hard for them to imagine their wife in pain or under anesthesia. I tell my patients this all the time: your husband's hesitation is usually rooted in concern for your safety, not judgment about your choice.

When I meet couples in consultations, I encourage partners to join us. It's powerful when a husband sees the before-and-after photos, or watches his wife's eyes light up as she tries on implant sizers and smiles for the first time in years. That's usually when it clicks for him—this isn't about someone else's approval. It's about her joy. And when he sees that joy, he's all in.

I've even had husbands become my biggest cheerleaders. They walk into follow-ups beaming. One told me, 'She hasn't stopped smiling since the surgery. It's like I got my wife back.' Moments like that never get old.

--Teamwork: A Family Affair

Every successful Mommy Makeover has one thing in common—support. Whether it's your partner, a friend, or your mom helping with meals and carpool, healing requires a team. And when you include your family in the preparation, it deepens connection instead of creating distance.

I often say that a Mommy Makeover is a family event. Everyone plays a part. You'll need extra help during recovery, but you'll also be teaching something valuable—how self-care creates a ripple effect of peace in the home. Your children, especially, will learn by watching you care for yourself.

--Talking With Your Kids

So how do you explain it to your kids? It depends on their age. For younger children, keep it simple: 'Mommy's having a special operation to help her feel better.' They don't need the details—they just need reassurance that you're okay and you'll be back to hugs soon.

I'll never forget one of my patients who told her eight-year-old daughter, 'Mommy's going to have tummy surgery.' When her daughter asked why, she said, 'Because the doctor said so.' The little girl shrugged and said, 'Okay.' Another mom told her boys she was having 'female surgery.' They groaned, yelled 'Gross!' and ran out of the room with plastic swords. And that was that.

For teens, honesty and example matter more. They're watching how you handle self-care and confidence. One mother told her 13-year-old daughter, 'As a mom, I've given my body to carry and raise children. Now I'm doing something to give back to myself.' That's a healthy model of self-respect—not vanity. It teaches your kids that caring for your body doesn't mean rejecting it—it means honoring it.

Your children don't need to understand every detail; they just need to feel your peace. When they see you confident and calm, they'll follow your lead.

Still, there's another layer of sensitivity here—especially when talking with children as they grow older. Some moms worry that by choosing surgery for themselves, they might accidentally send the message that their children will "need" to do the same someday.

I always remind my patients that how you frame your decision matters more than the decision itself. The message isn't, 'You should do this one day too.' It's, 'Mommy did this for Mommy.'

You can tell your kids, 'This was my choice, at my time, for reasons that felt right for me. You might make very different choices when you're older—and that's exactly how it should be.'

The goal isn't to create a standard to follow—it's to model thoughtfulness, honesty, and the courage to care for yourself in a healthy way.

Plastic surgery should never be something you feel pressured to do, and never something you should feel ashamed of considering. What I hope to show—through this book and through every patient story—is that beauty decisions are personal rights, not public debates.

If your children grow up understanding that confidence is self-defined, that self-care looks different for everyone, and that true strength lies in making choices aligned with your own values—they'll already have inherited the most beautiful part of your example.

--Talking With Family and Friends

Now, let's talk about everyone else—the people who might have opinions you didn't ask for. Telling family or friends about your decision can stir up mixed reactions. Some will cheer you on. Others might question your choice. That's okay. Remember, you're not asking for their approval—you're sharing something meaningful because you value connection.

Start with those who will be supportive. Use those first conversations as practice runs. If someone reacts negatively, remind yourself that their reaction says more about them than about you. You might even compare it to naming a baby—everyone has an opinion, but you're the one who lives with the result.

Sometimes resistance comes from older generations. They might say, 'Well, I never had surgery and I turned out fine.' That's true—and it's also true that times have changed. Plastic surgery today isn't about excess—it's about alignment. It's about restoring confidence, not chasing perfection. You're not becoming someone new. You're returning to yourself.

--The Compassionate Conversation Framework

When discussing your decision, lead with your feelings, not your defenses. Here's a framework I often share with patients: use an *I Statement.*

Example: 'I want to feel confident again so I can show up as my best self for our family.'

Example: 'I want to feel comfortable in my body so I can enjoy intimacy again without holding back.'

Example: 'I want to feel proud of my reflection so I can stop hiding in photos and start celebrating memories again.'

When you speak from this place, no one can argue with your truth. You're not making a case—you're sharing your heart.

The I Statement Exercise

Take a few minutes and write your own. Fill in the blanks:

I want to feel ______________________ **so I can show up as** ______________________.

Let it be honest. Let it be yours. Maybe it's confident. Maybe it's peaceful. Maybe it's joyful. Whatever the words, they're your compass. They remind you—and anyone who loves you—why this journey matters.

Because at its core, a Mommy Makeover isn't about seeking permission. It's about reconnecting—with your partner, your family, your reflection, and the woman you've always been.

Nashville Natural Notes-Practical wisdom from the consultation room

A Mommy Makeover isn't about seeking permission. It's about reconnecting—with your partner, your family, your reflection, and the woman you've always been.

And when you speak your truth clearly, the conversations that follow don't just change minds—they change hearts.

Plastic surgery should never be something you feel pressured to do, and never something you should feel ashamed of considering. What I hope to show—through this book and through every patient story—is that beauty decisions are personal rights, not public debates.

If your children grow up understanding that confidence is self-defined, that self-care looks different for everyone, and that true strength lies in making choices aligned with your own values—they'll already have inherited the most beautiful part of your example.

CHAPTER 8 Choosing the Right Surgeon for Your Soul and Skin

"Credentials matter—but connection matters more."

The most expensive mistake isn't the wrong operation—it's the wrong surgeon.

Every woman researching a Mommy Makeover eventually faces this truth: the person behind the scalpel matters as much as the procedure itself. The wrong fit can leave you feeling unseen or unfulfilled, even if the technical result looks perfect.

The right fit, however, changes everything.

This chapter is about choosing your surgeon—not just your surgery.

Credentials Are the Foundation, Not the Finish Line

Let's start with the basics. Many women are surprised to learn there's a difference between a *cosmetic surgeon* and a *board-certified plastic surgeon.* While every plastic surgeon performs cosmetic surgery, not every cosmetic surgeon is a plastic surgeon.

According to the American Board of Plastic Surgery (ABPS), becoming board-certified requires a minimum of five years of residency training in all areas of surgery, with at least two years devoted entirely to plastic surgery. Then come the rigorous written and oral exams—hundreds of questions, and panels of experienced surgeons reviewing every detail of your work to ensure it meets the highest standards of safety and ethics.

By contrast, cosmetic surgeons may come from virtually any medical background—OB/GYN, dermatology, even family medicine or emergency medicine—and sometimes complete only a weekend course before adding "cosmetic" to their title.

Why does that matter? Because you deserve someone who has trained for years to understand both the *art* and the *anatomy* of transformation.

As I often tell my patients:

"You wouldn't ask me to deliver your baby, and you shouldn't ask your obstetrician to do your tummy tuck."

Credentials ensure competence—but they don't guarantee chemistry.

Beyond Test Scores — Finding a Surgeon Who Sees You

Even after you've verified the letters after someone's name, you're not done. Credentials are the *starting line*, not the finish line.

When choosing your surgeon, look for three things:

1. Competence — Verify training, experience, and artistry. Review their before-and-after photos, and look for patients who share your body type and goals.

2. Character — Pay attention to how they speak *to you,* not *at you.* Do they listen more than they talk? Do they explain procedures clearly, without jargon or pressure?

3. Chemistry — Ask yourself: *Do I feel rushed or respected? Seen or processed?*

Surgery is intimate work. You deserve someone who treats you like family, not like a file number.

If you don't feel a connection, keep looking. The right surgeon will make you feel at ease, informed, and empowered. The wrong one will leave you second-guessing yourself before you've even scheduled your surgery.

Relationship Driven Plastic Surgery — Our Philosophy

At Music City Plastic Surgery, we don't just restore bodies; we rebuild confidence and connection.

I call this **Relationship Driven Plastic Surgery** — the belief that every transformation begins with trust.

My mission has always been to treat every woman as I would want my wife or mother to be treated—with dignity, compassion, honesty, and excellence.

It's about creating relationships, not transactions; transformation, not turnover.

Our Core Values

Unequivocal Excellence to Exceed Expectations

We don't settle for "good enough." Every step of your journey—from consultation to follow-up—is designed to surpass what you imagined possible.

Patient WOW Experience

Every interaction should make you say *"Wow."* From the first phone call to your one-year follow-up, we want you to feel seen, celebrated, and supported.

Anticipate and Answer the Unasked Questions

We believe the best care happens before anxiety begins. Our team is trained to educate, reassure, and prepare you long before worry has a chance to grow.

Because of our experience, we understand concerns before they're voiced—and we address them before they arise.

Authenticity & Integrity

We do what's right even when no one is looking. Honesty, humility, and transparency are nonnegotiable. We don't "sell" procedures—we guide decisions. If a procedure is not warranted for you or your situation, I will tell you plainly. I'd rather treat you right, than hustle you for a quick buck.

These aren't marketing slogans. They're the compass points that guide every choice we make as a team.

What Makes Us Different

We're proud to offer one of the **most comprehensive consultation processes in Nashville, maybe in the U.S.**—a full hour (or more) dedicated to understanding you, not rushing you through a checklist.

And our commitment doesn't end when the sutures dissolve. We provide **one of the longest follow-up processes in the country—up to a full year of care**—because your healing doesn't end at six weeks, and neither does our responsibility.

When you step into our office, you're not greeted with a clipboard and a backless gown.

You're offered a soft, floor-length spa robe that closes in the front—a small but powerful symbol that you're a person first, not a procedure.

The Consultation Experience

I've never believed in the "five-minute consult."

Your first appointment is where we begin to understand not only your *goals* but your *motives.*

I want to know what's held you back, what excites you about change, and what success will feel like when you see it in the mirror.

During our time together, we talk, we measure, we plan.

I might show you in the mirror how we'll reshape your silhouette, where your new contours will appear, and how your reflection will align with the woman you already are on the inside.

The goal isn't to push a certain procedure—it's to craft a plan that honors both your anatomy and your identity.

That takes time. That takes trust.

Nashville Natural Notes–Practical wisdom from the consultation room

Choosing the Right Relationship

At the end of the day, you're not just choosing a surgeon.

You're choosing a relationship.

You're choosing who will hold your story, your body, and your trust.

The right surgeon doesn't see flaws to fix—they see potential waiting to be uncovered.

They don't sculpt vanity; they help you rediscover your vitality.

"Credentials may open the door—but connection keeps you safe inside it."

Activity: 10 Questions to Ask Before You Commit

Before scheduling your surgery, take time to ask these—and trust how the answers *feel*, not just how they sound.

1. Is your surgeon board-certified by the American Board of Plastic Surgery (ABPS)?
2. How many Mommy Makeovers have they performed in the past year?
3. Do they personally perform all parts of your surgery?
4. What is their plan for post-op follow-up and emergencies?
5. How do they handle complications or revisions?
6. How long will they follow your healing journey?
7. What is their philosophy of beauty and confidence?
8. How do you feel in their office—heard or hurried?
9. What do their past patients say about their experience?
10. Do you trust them with your safety *and* your story?

Because this isn't just surgery—it's a relationship that shapes your reflection, your confidence, and your story for years to come.

Closing Reflection

Choosing your surgeon is the moment your journey turns from research to trust.

The right surgeon will not only understand your anatomy—but your *why.*

When those two align, transformation happens on every level: body, mind, and soul.

That's not just good surgery.

That's Relationship Driven Plastic Surgery.

CHAPTER 9
Under the Knife, Into the Light

What really happens in the OR — the art behind the science.

For most moms, the hardest part of surgery isn't the incision—it's the surrender.

You're used to being the one who holds everything together—the planner, the caretaker, the protector.

But surgery asks you to do the unthinkable: to let go, to lie down, to trust.

And I understand how hard that is—not just as a surgeon, but as a husband and a father.

I've been on the other side of things—after performing my wife's own Mommy Makeover surgery—my stomach tight, praying for her safe recovery.

I know what it means to need her here—for our family, for our kids, for me. That day, I understood —on the deepest level—what it means to hold someone's world in your hands.

It humbled me.

Because every woman who trusts me in that operating room is someone's mother, someone's wife, someone's daughter. Every patient who enters into my operating room deserves that same level of devotion, reverence, and care.

Each time I stand at the scrub sink, I pause for a silent prayer.

I ask God to steady my mind and hands, to guide my team, and to protect the patient who has entrusted me with her body and her spirit.

I thank Him for the opportunity to serve—and for the privilege of helping someone rediscover herself.

I whisper a version of these same words every single time:

"Lord, please be with us in this room. Guide my decisions and my hands. Keep her safe and protect her. Allow me to bring the desired result forth with care and precision. Help me do my part to heal not just what is seen, but what is unseen."

That quiet prayer is my moment of surrender—just as you, in trusting me, are offering yours.

The Fear Factor: Understanding the Surrender

Every mom I've ever operated on has had some version of the same thought:

"What if I don't wake up?"

And that thought carries weight—because it's not rooted in vanity; it's rooted in love. Moms aren't afraid for themselves. They're afraid for everyone who needs them.

That's why I **never** take your decision lightly. You're not just choosing a procedure. You're choosing trust. You're choosing to believe that someone else will protect what you value most—your life, your body, your ability to be there for your family.

As a father of four, I honor that fear. I acknowledge it. I see the guilt that sometimes comes with it—this whisper that says, *"What if something happens to me and it's my fault, because this was elective?"* That guilt is powerful. And I want you to know, I understand it completely.

It's also why I approach every case with this thought:

"This is someone's somebody."

That sacred responsibility shapes everything I do. I often remind my patients with a bit of humor:

"After surgery, I don't just want you to look beautiful—I want you to be alive and beautiful."

I want your kids, your spouse, and your family to have you around for a long, long time.

And the truth is—because we only operate on healthy, carefully screened patients—this surgery *is* happy, healthy medicine. It's not "have to" surgery; it's "want to" surgery. That difference matters. You're choosing joy, not chasing survival. And that's worth celebrating.

Nashville Natural Notes-Practical wisdom from the consultation room

You're not just choosing a procedure.

You're choosing trust.

You're choosing to believe that someone else will protect what you value most—your life, your body, your ability to be there for your family.

Transparency: What Really Happens in the OR

When you arrive at our surgery center, you'll notice immediately—it doesn't feel like a hospital. No one calls your name from behind a plastic divider for everyone in the waiting room to hear. There's no smell of antiseptics or echo of hurried footsteps.

Instead, you'll see familiar faces from our clinic—nurses and staff who already know you by name, who've walked beside you through your consultations and your pre-op visits. You'll notice the calm. The warmth. The privacy. That's not an accident.

We intentionally schedule one patient at a time so that when you arrive, you are our only focus. The entire environment is built for serenity—private rooms with closing doors instead of thin curtains, warm lighting, soft voices, and gentle movements. Our team anticipates what you'll need before you have to ask.

Your preoperative booklet, which you'll already have read at home, answers nearly every question we know might arise. The goal is to replace uncertainty with understanding. Because when anxiety meets clarity, fear starts to lose its grip.

The People Behind the Masks

Every member of my surgical team is handpicked—not just for their technical skill but for their heart. They are nurses, anesthesia providers, and techs who live the mantra of **Relationship Driven Plastic Surgery.**

They know what it's like to be vulnerable, to hand your body over to someone else's care. Many have been patients themselves. And that's why they treat every woman not as a "case," but as a person worthy of gentleness, dignity, and respect.

We talk about this as a team often: that compassion doesn't clock out when anesthesia begins. Even when you're asleep, you're never just a body—we see you as a story.

A Walk Through the Room

When it's time for surgery, you'll be gently rolled down the hall from your private pre-op room. You'll notice the air feels cooler—that's to maintain sterility and to keep us alert. The bright lights may surprise you at first, but everything is designed for one reason: your safety.

The room hums softly, like an orchestra warming up. Everyone knows their part. No chaos, no shouting, no rush—just a rhythm of calm precision.

Your anesthesia team will place a small oxygen mask over your face. It smells a little like a new shower curtain. They'll tell you to take a few slow breaths. Some patients remember counting down from 100. Most don't make it past 97 before drifting peacefully to sleep.

That's the last thing you'll remember until you wake up, safe and warm, with the surgery complete.

The Art Behind the Science

To the outside world, surgery looks purely mechanical—machines, monitors, measurements. But beneath that precision lies art.

Every incision is mapped and measured, but the beauty is in the nuance—the angle of a line, the subtlety of a curve, the balance between symmetry and softness. It's an orchestration of anatomy and intuition.

Plastic surgery, at its best, lives where science meets soul; where millimeters meet meaning, and every stitch tells a story.

Each operation is both technical and spiritual for me. Long before we ever step into the OR, I've visualized your surgery in my mind—where I'll place the incision, how your contours will look, how your posture will feel when you see yourself again.

By the time I'm operating, I'm simply bringing that vision to life.

And through it all, I feel God's presence guiding my hands—steadying them when precision is needed, softening them when grace is required.

The Awakening

The next thing you'll remember is waking up, blinking softly as your body adjusts. The first thought most women have is, *"Wait—is it already over?"*

Our nurses are right there beside you, wrapping you in warmth, adjusting your blankets, speaking gently as the anesthesia wears off. They'll help you get dressed, keep you comfortable, and ensure your safety before you leave.

And yes, this is the part of the day that gives us our share of funny stories. I've had patients wake up declaring their undying love for me—or cursing me out. I take neither personally, it's all part of a day's work. OK, maybe I take the positive accolades to heart a little bit. It does do my ego good.

Within an hour, you'll be ready to go home with your caregiver, where the real healing begins. And when you're ready, I'll see you again—the same face that greeted you that morning, now meeting you with pride and care in your first post-op visit.

Closing Reflection: Trust and Transformation

Surgery, in many ways, mirrors faith. You step into the unknown, surrender control, and trust that on the other side, there will be light.

My role is to earn that trust—to hold it gently, honor it completely, and carry it into every decision, every stitch, every prayer.

Because this work isn't just about transformation—it's about reverence.

You give me your trust, and I give you my hands.
Together, through faith and science,
we find your reflection waiting on the other side.

Visualization for Calm and Confidence

Find a quiet place. Sit or lie comfortably. Close your eyes.

Picture yourself walking through the doors of our surgery center. The air smells clean, the light is soft, and you're greeted by a friendly nurse who hands you a warm blanket. You recognize faces that make you feel safe.

You take a slow, steady breath.

Next, I greet you with a calm smile and say, "We're going to take great care of you." You feel peace begin to rise where fear once lived.

As you lie back, imagine the light above you—bright, but not harsh. It feels like sunrise through a window. That light surrounds you, holds you, and when you awaken, it's still there—only now, it shines from within.

"Remember: calm is contagious, and so is confidence."

CHAPTER 10

Healing Without Hustle

"Rest isn't weakness—it's medicine."

Most mothers I meet don't fear the surgery half as much as they fear the stillness that follows it.

You're used to being the doer.
The mover.
The picker-upper, the problem-solver, the keeper of all plates spinning.

But healing has a different rhythm.
It does not respond to hustle.
It requires surrender.

And in this chapter, I want to help you prepare for that surrender—not as a loss of control, but as a return to balance.

Because rest isn't a luxury.
Rest is medicine.

The Real Work of Recovery

"Healing isn't just physical — it's emotional rebirth."

If you're the typical Mommy Makeover patient, you're juggling:

Children.
A home.

Work.
A partner.
Schedules.
Meals.
A thousand invisible tasks.

And because you carry so much, when surgery enters the picture, your first instinct is guilt:

"I should be doing more."
"Everyone needs me."
"How can I step back now?"

But here is the truth:

Your family needs you healed more than they need you busy.

Healing is not passive.
It is intentional, restorative work—just quieter than the work you're used to.

This chapter is your permission to release the hustle, embrace the pause, and honor what your body is about to do.

Preparing For The Pause

Once you decide to move forward, we usually schedule surgery a few weeks out.
This time is not just for lab work, payments, and logistics.

It's for preparing your *heart.*

Most women underestimate how difficult the *mental* shift can be.
Not the surgery—not the pain—not the logistics.

But giving themselves permission to rest.

I want you to know this:

You deserve this time.
You are worth this healing.
And the world will wait while you mend.

Prepare your environment now so your mind can let go later:

- Lighten the calendar.
- Stock the fridge.
- Finish the laundry.
- Set out clothes for the kids.
- Organize carpools.
- Make the home tidy, calm, and ready for your return.

And once it's done?

Release it.

Perfection will not help you heal.
Surrender will.

Let It Go (Before You Lie Down)

No matter how well you prepare, recovery won't unfold like a Pinterest board.

Meals may not be gourmet.
The floor may not be spotless.

Your kids may wear the same outfit more than once.
Schedules may flex.

And that's okay.

As a father of four and a husband to another physician, trust me: life survives temporary disorder.
Your kids will actually be thrilled with pizza every night.
At our house, before we had our daughter, my sons and I would call it a "man's meal"—hot dogs, burgers, and exactly zero vegetables.

They think it's heaven.

Let them have their version of joy.
Let the house breathe.
Let yourself heal.

Outta Sight, Outta Mind (A Secret Weapon)

One of the best strategies I've ever seen moms use?

A recovery getaway.

A quiet hotel suite.
A recovery room.
A friend's peaceful guest room.

Somewhere away from:

- Crying toddlers
- Unfolded laundry
- Clattering dishes
- Toy explosions

- The chaos you're hardwired to fix

Distance isn't avoidance—it's *protection.*

If you can't see the mess, you can't be tempted to fix it.
If you can't hear the noise, you can rest in peace.

Sometimes the best gift you can give your healing body...
is silence.

Planning For Recovery

The timeline your body will thank you for.

Downtime is usually two to three weeks.
And for many moms, this is the hardest assignment they've ever been given.

Because if you rush your healing:

- Tummy tuck repairs can tear
- Implants can shift
- Scars can stretch
- Swelling worsens
- Pain increases
- Results can be compromised

Your body will tell you when you're pushing too soon.
I call it "reminder pain."
It's your body whispering:
"Slow down. I'm rebuilding."

Honor that whisper.

Nashville Natural Notes-Practical wisdom from the consultation room

Healing Is Part of the Result

Beautiful results don't just come from surgery.

They come from patience during recovery.

Walking, resting, and allowing the body time to heal are just as important as the procedure itself.

Choose Help That Feels Like Peace

During your first days, you *must* have an adult with you—someone gentle, supportive, and calm.

Choose people who bring peace, not pressure:

- A partner who is truly helpful
- A close friend
- A family member who understands boundaries
- A night nurse or private caregiver

Choose people who can see you vulnerable — groggy, emotional, messy — and love you through it without judgment.

This is sacred space.
Only the gentle belong here.

The Science of Stillness

Here's what most people don't know:

Your body heals best in calm.

Stillness is not the absence of activity—it is the environment in which the body regenerates:

- Collagen knits.
- Swelling decreases.
- Blood flow improves.
- Scar tissue softens.
- Nerves recalibrate.
- Muscles repair.
- Inflammation drops.

Stillness is not weakness.
It is wisdom written into your biology.

Healing Is A Verb

The emotional timeline no one talks about.

Recovery will test your patience.
Some days you will feel confident, strong, beautiful.
Other days you may feel swollen, discouraged, or emotional.

Nothing is wrong with you.
That is the rhythm of healing.

Comparison is the enemy of peace.
Do not compare your body, your scars, your swelling, or your timeline with anyone else.

Healing is not a race.
It's a relationship—with your body, with your patience, with your future self.

The Permission To Pause Checklist

Five Non-Negotiables for Recovery

1. Hydrate before caffeine.
2. Sleep before screens.
3. Walk gently, breathe deeply.
4. Nourish your body with intention.
5. Ask for help before you think you need it.

Healing is holy work. Treat it that way.

Activity: The "Why List"

Your emotional anchor for the journey ahead

Before surgery, take a moment to write down:

Three reasons you want this surgery.
Three ways you hope to feel afterward.

This becomes your compass.

During recovery, when impatience or doubt whispers, return to this list.
It will remind you of your truth.

Activity: The Pre-Op Gratitude Log

Preparing the heart for healing

For the next seven nights, write down:

Three things your body has carried you through — pregnancy, birth, the hard seasons, the beautiful moments, the sacrifices, the storms you didn't think you'd survive.

This is not about surgery.
This is about honoring the resilience already inside you.

Gratitude softens fear.
Fear softens resistance.
And softness prepares the heart for healing.

The Long Game Of Grace

Protecting your results. Protecting your peace.

Your Mommy Makeover is not a finish line.
It is a new beginning.

Genetics, gravity, lifestyle — they still matter.
But now you have a restored foundation.

Honor it with:

- Steady weight
- Consistent movement
- Nourishing food
- Hormonal awareness
- Emotional self-care

This isn't about perfection.
It's about partnership between you, your surgeon, and your healing body.

You didn't come this far to abandon yourself now.

Closing Reflection

Your body has healed others.
Now, it is your turn.

Rest without guilt.
Heal without hurry.
Recover without apology.

Stillness is not the pause between chapters —
it is the chapter where you return to yourself.

CHAPTER 11
The Emotional Curve of Change

"Transformation isn't a straight line—it's a roller coaster with dips, climbs, and breathtaking views you can't see from the ground."

Every woman imagines transformation as a clean upward rise. A steady climb. A predictable progression from decision → surgery → confidence.

But real transformation—the kind that touches identity, not just anatomy—isn't a staircase.

It's a roller coaster.

Not the wild, reckless kind with loose bolts and shaky rails. But the kind you choose to ride because you know the view at the top is worth the twists along the way.

There's the moment you get in line with excitement and anticipation. Then the moment your stomach drops and you wonder if you made a terrible mistake. Then the climb... the dips... the thrill... the fear... the laughter... the relief... the joy.

And most importantly:

You don't ride it because it's easy.
You ride it because you're headed somewhere beautiful.

This chapter is here to remind you that every turn has purpose.

The Night-Before Drop: When Fear Buckles the Seat Belt

Nearly every mom I operate on has *the moment*— the emotional drop before the climb.

It might happen the night before.
Or in the car on the way to the surgery center.
Or even lying on the operating table just before anesthesia.

The thoughts sound almost universal:

"Why am I doing this?"
"Should I be risking this?"
"My kids need me."
"Is this silly? Is this vain?"
"What if something happens?"

Let me tell you something with full sincerity:

This is the first dip on the roller coaster.
It's not a warning sign — it's a human sign.

These are all normal and expected reactions to undergoing something so personal and powerful in your life. We talk about it beforehand so *when,* and not *if,* this happens, you can better manage it. I encourage each mom to give herself some Grace as these emotions appear, to not dwell on to it or beat herself up for experiencing them.

The First Climb: When Logic and Love Battle for the Same Space

You remind yourself:

- You sacrificed your body for your children.
- You've earned the right to reclaim it.
- This surgery is safe.
- You're doing this thoughtfully, not impulsively.
- You're doing this for confidence, not attention.

But your mind is still chattering, because you're a mom.

Motherhood has rewired your brain to calculate risk on behalf of the people you love most in the world.

You're not crazy.
You're not selfish.
You're not unstable.

You're protective.

And yet, guilt tries to pull you back down the track.

So hear this clearly:

You are not choosing between your family and yourself.
You are choosing both — because a restored you is a stronger you.

The roller coaster climbs.

The Night-Before Tears

Lauren cried the night before surgery, afraid and guilty.
I reminded her:

"Feeling this way doesn't mean you're not ready. It means you're a mom."

Months later she told me that that moment was when she finally stepped back toward herself.

Her roller coaster had just begun.

THE MID-RIDE: When the Post-Op Emotions Swing Hard

Once the surgery is over, a new part of the ride begins.

You're tender.
You're swollen.
You're sore.
You're bandaged.
You're exhausted.
You're dependent (which most moms hate).

And suddenly, the emotional rails shift:

One moment:
"I'm so glad I did this."

Ten minutes later:
"What have I done?"

That's not inconsistency — that's physiology:

- Anesthesia residue

- Sleep disruption
- Hormonal shifts
- Medication effects
- Temporary loss of control
- A pause in your normal routines
- Body-image uncertainty during swelling
- Fear of the unknown
- And yes... impatience

Every mom riding this part of the roller coaster thinks she's the only one experiencing this.

You're not.

This is one of the most universal emotional patterns I've ever seen.

And the beautiful truth?

These dips usually come *right before* the breakthroughs.

The Day 3 Dip

Melissa called on day three, crying, convinced she'd made a mistake.
A week later she looked in the mirror and whispered,
"Okay... there you are."

Her dip wasn't failure.
It was healing in motion.

The Turning Point: When the Track Begins to Rise Again

It happens subtly:

A little less soreness.
A little less swelling.
A little more energy.
A glimpse in the mirror that feels... hopeful.
A shirt fitting differently.
A waistline returning.
A curve reappearing.

One day you turn slightly in the mirror —
and something clicks.

Recognition.
Relief.
Reclaiming.

This is the moment you realize:

"I'm coming back."

And the roller coaster starts to climb.

Not all at once — but one gentle click at a time.

This is where true transformation begins:

- Confidence rises
- Self-esteem returns
- Identity reconnects

- Intimacy rekindles
- Joy re-emerges

This part of the ride is worth every dip that came before it.

The First Glimpse

Twelve days after surgery, Hannah raised her garment, gasped, and whispered:
"That's me."
Not the stretched skin.
Not the years of exhaustion.
Her.
Her emotional curve had reached its rise.

The Light Moments: Humor on the Ride

Not every turn is heavy.

Some moments are unexpectedly joyful —
especially the ones fueled by anesthesia.

I've seen the most reserved moms become comedians when they wake up.

Laughter, too, is part of healing.

The Post-Op Comedy Hour

Jessica woke up telling the nurse she was beautiful.
She sang about how much she loved me.
Then loudly asked her husband:

"Are my breasts perky yet?"

She was mortified later.
But healing sometimes comes wrapped in joy — and laughter.

The Shared Ride: When Transformation Lifts a Family

A Mommy Makeover doesn't just touch the woman — it touches the household.

Some partners worry.
Some step up.
Some deepen their empathy.
Some see their wives shine again for the first time in years.

And sometimes, the emotional curve becomes a shared journey.

The Husband Who Finally Understood

"In my view, she didn't need surgery," he said.
"But I missed the way she lit up."

He helped her bathe, held her hand, made her soup.
At follow-up he said to me:
"Thank you for giving my wife back to herself."

Sometimes the roller coaster lifts an entire family.

Understanding The Emotional Roller Coaster

Although it's difficult to point to a single exact cause, many factors exist to build this emotional roller coaster. Surgery is a significant physical stress to your body, general anesthesia is used, narcotic pain medications are prescribed, and steroids may be used—all of which can throw off your hormone balances. Pain may interfere with sleeping and deplete your body's reserves, leaving you feeling tired and worn down. I believe you heal more quickly when you are not in pain because your body devotes the resources to healing and not fighting pain, so I encourage use of the pain medications, at least in the first few days. However, the anesthesia and pain medications can also alter sleep patterns. As any mom remembers from the early times of her children's lives, life becomes a lot more difficult when you are lacking sleep.

Most moms tend to be dynamic individuals, often "going" at all times. The elevated endorphins they are used to having from frequent workouts and high activity levels are reduced or nonexistent in the recovery phase, when Mom has to be uncharacteristically still. Many moms have difficulty in this unstructured healing time and get antsy to do something.

Stress has a *huge* role in how you deal with the postoperative period. We already mentioned the physical stress of surgery, but the mental stress of the impending surgery, and then waiting for the final outcome, play into your emotions as well.

Often with surgery you may look worse before you look better. Seeing the swelling, bruising, and temporarily raised or reddened scars may leave Mom second-guessing why she voluntarily chose this. Anxiety works negatively in this situation. Anxiety about the results, about taking time for yourself, about being so behind in terms of your "job" as mom (the house is a mess, the kids are out of control, etc.), about being alone to fend for yourself if your husband has returned to work, about returning to your outside- the-house job sooner than you may feel ready for ... the list can go on and on.

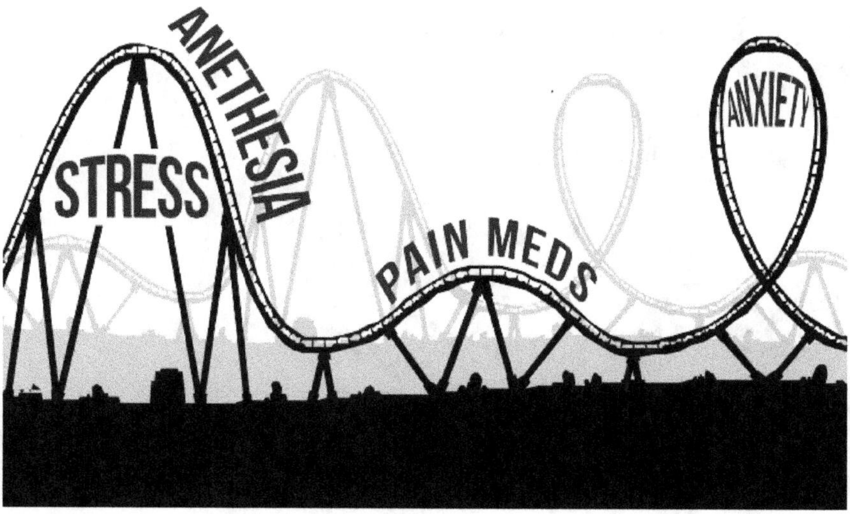

Putting The Brakes On The Emotional Roller Coaster

Here's how you protect your heart and your healing:

1. Get outside

Sunlight is medicine.

2. Shower

Women tell me they feel "human again" after the first one.

3. Eat in color

Protein and produce speed healing.

4. Avoid emotional toxins

Limit negativity during recovery.
Invite only safe, supportive people into your space.

5. See me if you're anxious

Part of my job is to reassure you.
I don't consider it a burden — it's a privilege.

6. Trust the timeline

Healing is not instant.
It is a sequence — a choreography.

And when impatience hits (and it will), tell yourself:

"I'm not stuck. I'm mid-ride."

Remember the time frame for healing from surgery. Many times, full results are not appreciated for a few months. Give your body the chance to heal before you second-guess your decisions. We'll discuss the specifics of each procedure in the following chapters so you will be well prepared and informed when it's time for your surgery.

Activity: Your Confidence Curve

On a sheet of paper, draw a wavy line — a roller coaster track.

Each day or week, mark:

- Your mood
- Your confidence
- Your energy
- Your body-image thoughts

This helps you see:

- How normal the dips are

- How steady the rises become
- How transformation happens gradually, not instantly

And the most powerful part?

When you look back, you'll see the truth:

You were rising long before you realized you were rising.

Closing Reflection

You didn't choose this journey because it was simple.
You chose it because you were ready for a new chapter.

And like every great ride, it has turns you don't expect,
moments that lift your stomach,
and views that take your breath away.

The emotional roller coaster isn't a sign you should get off.

It's the evidence you're on your way somewhere beautiful.

CHAPTER 12

The Ripple Effect of Confidence

"When a mother rises, the whole family rises with her."

Confidence is never selfish.
It is never solitary.
And it is never contained.

When a mother feels beautiful again—not for the world, but for *herself*—the change radiates outward in ways few people expect.

It softens her tone.
Brightens her presence.
Lifts her posture.
Reawakens her joy.

Confidence is contagious.

And in a family, the mother is often the epicenter of that contagion.

This chapter isn't about contour lines or incision placement.
It's about what happens **after**—when the internal shift becomes an external blessing for everyone she loves.

The Lie Society Tells Moms

Society loves to shame women with two contradictory messages:

- "Bounce back immediately after birth."
- "But don't you dare consider surgery—you should love your 'battle scars.'"

It's a trap women aren't meant to escape.

If a mom struggles with her postpartum body, she's told to accept it.
If she wants to improve it, she's told she's vain.
If she invests in herself, she's told she's selfish.

But here is what I've seen after thousands of surgeries:

A confident mother is a more present, patient, connected mother.

Not because her waist is smaller.
Not because her breasts are lifted.
Not because society approves.

But because she sees herself again—
and when a woman reconnects with herself, she reconnects with everyone around her.

This isn't vanity.
This is restoration.

And restoration always ripples.

The Inner Circle Ripples

The Spouse Ripple

A husband once sat in my office, tears in his eyes, holding his wife's hand as she admired herself at her first post-op appointment.

He whispered:

**"I didn't fall in love with your body.
I fell in love with your joy.
And I've missed this version of you."**

Her transformation wasn't about becoming someone new.
It was about him seeing the woman he married rise back to the surface.

Confidence restored intimacy — not just physically, but emotionally.

Marriage Ripple Story: *The Marriage That Found Its Spark Again*

Emily had been married fifteen years. She loved her husband deeply, but she felt disconnected from the woman she once was.

After her Mommy Makeover, her husband kept quietly studying her — not her body, but her *joy* returning.
One day, while folding laundry, he said:

**"You laugh differently now.
I didn't realize how long it's been since I heard that sound."**

Their intimacy rekindled not because her body changed,
but because she felt like herself again.

Confidence gave their marriage room to breathe — and to blossom again.

Recently, I had a patient who came back in a year or two after her surgery remark about how it actually took her a while to get used to her new figure, to think of herself as this newer version when looking in the mirror. We see this a lot with moms, especially those who had significant weight gain with pregnancy or with multiple pregnancies. It almost seems a new identity had been created. This has to get 'unlearned' after surgery, and the mom reminded of who she still is. This can take a bit of time as often the mom equates the overhang, the mom pooch, as a battle scar of becoming a mom. She's still the same person she was prior; she just helped grow another human inside her. I encourage her to remember who she is when she looks in the mirror.

On one occasion, a patient's husband pulled me aside after a visit. A bit sheepish, he admitted he also needed time to adjust. Though they'd been married for over a decade, he said it felt like seeing the woman he first fell in love with again. With time, they both settled into this restored sense of identity— a confident woman who is also a mom.

The Children Ripple

A mom once told me:

"My daughter said, 'Mommy, you smile more now.'"

Children internalize their parents' emotions long before they understand them.
When a mother feels weighed down—emotionally or physically—her children sense it.

But when she feels lighter, freer, more aligned?

Her children change too:

- calmer mornings
- more patience
- more energy
- more joy
- more confidence modeled for them

Confidence changes parenting.
Not because of appearance —
but because confidence allows moms to show up fully present.

Daughter Ripple Story: *The Daughter Who Found Her Own Confidence*

One patient brought her daughter to every post-op visit so she could witness the process.
By the third visit, the girl stood taller, asked questions, and smiled more.

At the final appointment, she said:

"Mom... you seem more like you again."

Later she whispered to me:

"My mom is brave."

A daughter raised by a confident mother learns self-respect, self-care, and self-worth — not through lectures, but through example.

Son Ripple Story: *The Son Who Finally Understood*

A teenage boy once watched quietly at his mom's follow-up visit, pretending not to care.
But after seeing her relax and smile, he told her:

"You look really happy.
I didn't know how much this meant to you."

He carried her purse out of the office.
At home, he was gentler, more helpful, more aware.

He didn't change because her body changed —
he changed because he saw his mom's spirit lift.

A son who sees his mother honor herself grows into a man who honors women.

The Outer Circle Ripples

The Friend Ripple

A group of women once visited saying:

"She went first — now it's our turn."

When one mother steps into confidence, her friends see possibility.

Confidence is magnetic.
It inspires.
It liberates.

It expands what other women believe is available to them.

The Professional Ripple

Confidence doesn't stay at home —
it walks into the office.

Some women start:

- speaking up
- asking for promotions
- setting boundaries
- commanding rooms
- leading with calm dignity

This isn't ego. It's alignment.

When insecurity is no longer draining their energy, their potential rises.

The Promotion She Finally Asked For

Kara was brilliant but hesitant.
She hid her postpartum body in loose clothes and avoided leadership opportunities.

After her Mommy Makeover, she told me:

**"It's not that I look different at work.
It's that I *show up* differently."**

She asked for — and received — a promotion she'd avoided for years.

Her body didn't change her career.
Her confidence did.

The Extended Ripples: The Legacy Circle

This ripple might be the most powerful:

The generational shift.

A confident mother teaches:

- Self-care is not selfish
- Confidence is allowed
- Resilience is modeled
- Beauty is multifaceted
- Womanhood is strong, not fragile

Her daughters learn to love themselves.
Her sons learn to respect women.

This isn't cosmetic.

This is legacy work.

Activity: The Confidence Ripple Map

On a blank page:

1. Write your name in the center.
2. Draw circles radiating outward.
3. Label them:

- Spouse
- Children

- Friends
- Family
- Workplace
- Community
- Self

4. For each, write one sentence:
   "What changes when I feel whole again?"

You'll see that confidence never stays in one place.
It always travels.

Closing Reflection

You did not choose this journey to become someone new.

You chose it to come home to yourself —
and coming home to yourself lifts everyone in your orbit.

Never underestimate the quiet, extraordinary power
of a confident mother.

Because when she rises,
the world around her rises too.

CHAPTER 13
Uncovering the Hidden You

"This isn't a makeover — it's a homecoming."

There is a moment — sometimes whispered, sometimes sudden — when a woman looks at her reflection and realizes:

"I'm back."

Not the pre-baby version of herself.
Not the younger version.
Not the airbrushed, edited, impossible version.

But the truest version.
The one she feared was gone... but was only hidden beneath years of sacrifice, exhaustion, and self-forgetting.

A Mommy Makeover doesn't create someone new.
It removes the layers — physical, emotional, and spiritual — that have covered her for too long.

This chapter is about **staying connected** to the woman you've uncovered.

Because confidence is not a moment.
It is a practice.
A relationship.
A way of living.

The Fear That Beauty Fades

Every patient eventually asks some version of the same quiet question:

"Will these results last?"
"Will I still feel this confident years from now?"
"What if it slips away again?"

And I always answer:

Your beauty wasn't created in surgery.
It was *revealed.*
And what is revealed can always be remembered.

Yes, gravity continues its pull.
Yes, genetics leave their fingerprints.
Yes, time has its say.

But beauty that comes from alignment —
from peace, from clarity, from self-respect, from restored identity —
doesn't fade with the mirror.

It deepens.

Because what you've truly uncovered isn't a contour.
It's a connection.

A highly accomplished patient once shared that when people looked at her, she assumed it was for negative reasons tied to her appearance. After surgery, that shifted. Now when she stands at a podium, she knows the attention is for her ideas and expertise. Free from the distraction of negative body thoughts, she focuses better, stands taller, and delivers her message with greater impact.

The Long View: Sustaining The Transformation

Plastic surgery is not magic — it's collaboration.
I sculpt, you heal, and together we protect the results.

No matter how skilled your surgeon, no result is immune to time. But your habits, your environment, and your mindset hold tremendous power.

Here's what matters most long-term:

1. Honor your body with consistency, not perfection.

Weight stability is key not just for your results, but for your overall well-being.

2. Move because you love yourself, not because you're correcting yourself.

Exercise isn't punishment — it's devotion.

3. Feed your body with what gives it energy, clarity, and resilience.

Nutrition is one of the quiet protectors of beauty.

4. Protect your skin the way you protect your children.

Sunscreen. Hydration. Quality skincare.
Your skin is your lifelong garment — treat it gently.

5. Watch for emotional erosion.

Stress, guilt, caretaking overload — these can undo confidence faster than gravity can.

Sustaining beauty is not the pursuit of flawlessness.
It is the practice of gratitude.

Gratitude for the body that carried children.
Gratitude for the courage to reclaim it.
Gratitude for the resilience you now wear.

Gratitude is the anchor that keeps the "hidden you" from disappearing again.

The Spiritual Dimension of Sustained Beauty

Every time I scrub in for surgery, I say a silent prayer:

"Lord, please be with us in this room
Guard my decisions and my hands.
Keep her safe and protect her.
Allow me to bring the desired result forth with care and precision. Help me do my part to heal not just what is seen, but what is unseen."

But your long-term healing — the years after surgery —
that is where *your* prayer continues.

Self-care, rest, boundaries, nourishment —
these become acts of worship.
Acts of gratitude.
Acts of stewardship of the body God has entrusted to you.

Your beauty — the true beauty —
is sustained by how you honor your wholeness.

Not once.
But continually.

The Real Secret: Confidence Grows With Use

Confidence isn't like a candle that burns down.
It's a fire that grows when it's fed.

Use it.

Wear that dress.
Take that photo.
Book that trip.
Say yes to the date night.
Say no to the things that drain you.
Put your name in rooms where you belong.
Take up space without apology.

Your makeover uncovered the woman who was always meant to lead your life —
not hide behind it.

Let her live in the open.

Let me tell you about Kathryn. Physically, her journey had been grueling. During her pregnancy with her youngest, she developed toxemia and gained nearly 100 pounds. For four years, she fought back with a trainer and a disciplined diet, losing the weight but finding herself left with a body she didn't recognize. Her abdominal muscles had separated, creating a shape that no amount of crunches could fix, and her breasts were heavy and sagging, causing back and neck pain that interfered with her daily life. We decided on a comprehensive approach:

a breast lift/reduction, small implants, alongside the tummy tuck and muscle repair.

On the morning of surgery, she was surprisingly calm. But as I was making my pre-operative markings, she looked at me and said, "Just please make me beautiful." I stopped, looked her in the eye, and told her the truth: "You are already beautiful. I'm just going to enhance what you have."

Her recovery was remarkable—she was back to work in just twelve days. But the most profound change wasn't the physical one, though she went from a triple D to a perky C and achieved a flat stomach. The real transformation was mental. She went from feeling self-conscious and guilty to feeling worthy and deserving. Her confidence skyrocketed from a four to a ten. She told me she finally felt like her outside matched the strength she had always carried on the inside.

The Hidden You Was Never Really Lost

When you look back someday, I want you to see this truth clearly:

You didn't "get your body back."
You didn't "fix" yourself.
You didn't remake who you were.

You *returned* to who you were always becoming.

That is the real makeover.
That is the homecoming.

Activity: Your Confidence Manifesto

This is the final exercise of your journey —
a declaration, a promise, and a compass.

On a fresh page, write these words at the top:

"My Confidence Manifesto"

Then answer:

1. **Who am I now that I've uncovered myself again?**
2. **What do I promise to never apologize for again?**
3. **What habits will I carry forward to honor this transformation?**
4. **How will I protect my peace, my joy, and my confidence?**
5. **What will I teach my children about self-respect and beauty?**

Sign it.
Date it.
Keep it in a drawer, a Bible, a journal, or even your nightstand.

This is not a contract with perfection —
it is a covenant with yourself.

Closing Reflection

You came into this journey feeling hidden, stretched thin, pulled in every direction.
But now — standing here, grounded in your own reflection again — you know something sacred:

You were never lost.
Just waiting to be uncovered.

Your homecoming is not the end of the story.
It is the beginning of the life you were always meant to live.

Welcome home.

PART III
REBUILDING BEAUTIFUL: THE SURGICAL PROCEDURES

Inside the tools, techniques, and truths of transformation.

CHAPTER 14

Layered: The Invisible Map of the Post-Baby Body

The Truth About Layers, Luck, and the GLP-1 Revolution

If you've ever looked at your body and thought, *"Why won't this part respond?"*—

this chapter is for you.

Because the truth is, you're not failing.
You're not undisciplined.
And you're certainly not alone.

You're layered.

The Problem

Why Effort Doesn't Always Equal Outcome

One of the most frustrating things I hear from patients—especially mothers—is this:

"I eat well. I try to exercise. I've done what I can. And still... this won't move."

That frustration isn't imagined. It's biological.

Not all fat behaves the same way, and not all fat responds to effort equally. Hormones, metabolism, stress, sleep deprivation, pregnancy, age, medications, and simple genetics all play a role in where fat settles—and whether it's willing to leave.

To understand your options, you first need to understand **what kind of fat you're dealing with**.

Superficial vs. Visceral Fat

What You Can Pinch—and What You Can't

The superficial fat is the area that can be pinched directly below the skin when you do the "pinch an inch test" on your belly. The visceral fat is deeper and is often the unhealthy portion.

I like to start this conversation using men as examples—not because they're the focus of this book, but because their fat distribution is easier to visualize.

Visceral Fat: The Inside Layer

Most men tend to store fat **deep**, underneath the muscle layer, wrapped around the organs. This is called **visceral fat**.

Picture the classic barrel-chested or barrel-bellied man. When you push on his abdomen, there's very little "give" before you hit muscle. That firmness isn't strength—it's pressure from within.

Visceral fat pushes outward, increasing waist circumference and placing strain on the heart, liver, and metabolic system. It's why a waist circumference over 40 inches in men is strongly associated with increased morbidity and mortality.

This type of fat is **NOT surgically removable**. Historically, the only ways to reduce it were diet, exercise, and significant lifestyle change. Now things are different...read on to discover what.

Superficial Fat: The Outer Layer

Women, on the other hand, are biologically designed to carry more fat **superficially**—the layer just beneath the skin. This is the fat you can pinch. The fat that settles in the abdomen, hips, thighs, arms, and back.

This difference is one reason plastic surgeons tend to have very good relationships with women—we can help with what they carry.

That said, many women—especially after pregnancy or weight gain—carry **both** types of fat. And that distinction matters more than most people realize.

Why This Matters for Surgery

The Beach Ball Analogy

When I evaluate someone for body contouring, it's not just how much skin is loose that is important—it's also how much pressure exists underneath it.

Imagine I'm trying to button my suit jacket over a beach ball.

No matter how much fabric I have, there's a limit to how much I can tighten things down before the pressure pushes back. The human body works the same way.

Visceral fat lives inside the abdominal cavity, and that space can only compress so much before it presses against the spine and back of the body. If that internal pressure is high, it limits:

- How much I can tighten a waistline
- How effectively I can repair a diastasis recti
- Whether a tummy tuck will actually improve projection

In contrast, when visceral fat is reduced—through lifestyle change, medication, or surgical weight loss like gastric banding or gastric bypass—the success achieved in tightening this area is significantly increased.

This is why some patients are better served by **weight reduction first**, and others by **surgery now**. It's not about judgment. It's about physics.

The Truth Behind "Abs Are Made in the Kitchen"

You've probably heard the phrase. And while it's not wrong, it's incomplete.

What it ignores is real life.

With Kids.
Sleep Deprivation.
Breastfeeding.
Work.

The difficulty in planning, the truth that Mom is always last and typically only gets to eat a few bites of whatever is within an easy grasp. And with exercise, the logistical challenges of what to do with the kids, feeling tired because you were up all night breastfeeding or with a sick child, etc. etc. come into play.

I understand that. I see it every day.

What I share with patients—gently, honestly—is this:

The lower the visceral fat, the higher the potentials for surgical success.

That knowledge isn't meant to discourage you.
It's meant to empower you.

The Solution

Pulling Back the Curtain on GLP-1 Medications

If diet and exercise once felt like the only path—and an exhausting one at that—there is now another option that has changed the landscape entirely.

GLP-1 medications.

Think of them as a quiet recalibration rather than a shortcut.

Taken as a once-weekly injection or daily oral option, these GLP-1's (Glucagon-Like Peptide-1's) medications help you feel full longer, reduce "food noise," slow stomach emptying, signaling fullness to the brain and gently lower calorie intake. Over time, this leads to meaningful, sustained weight loss—often beginning after the second or third month.

For many patients, this feels almost mythical.

I sometimes joke that I feel like the Wizard of Oz when patients ask me for the secret—because for years, the answer was sacrifice without guarantee. Now, we finally have a tool that helps the body cooperate.

But unlike the Wizard, I don't hide behind a curtain.

These medications work by changing physiology—not willpower. And for patients with conditions like PCOS (poly cystic ovarian syndrome), hypothyroidism, diabetes, or decades of failed dieting, they can be genuinely life-changing.

The Tradeoffs—and the Truth

GLP-1s aren't magic without responsibility.

Potential side effects include nausea, dehydration, muscle loss, and—rarely—more serious complications. We mitigate these with:

- Hydration
- Adequate protein intake
- Strength training
- Gradual dose escalation
- Coaching and education

Most patients tolerate the adjustment period well, especially when they understand that the discomfort is temporary and the benefit is long-term.

And then there's the part no one talks about openly:

Rapid or significant weight loss can leave behind **excess skin**—the overstretched rubber band effect. This is where terms like "Ozempic belly", "Ozempic breast" or "Ozempic labia" come from.

This isn't failure.
It's physics.

And it's exactly where body contouring enters the conversation—not as vanity, but as completion.

Where Plastic Surgery Fits In

Not First. And Maybe Not Last.

Plastic surgery doesn't replace weight loss.
It honors it.

Once weight stabilizes, we can remove excess skin, tighten what remains, and restore proportion—so your outside finally matches the work you've done on the inside. This can be done at the end, but can also be performed when a patient reaches a plateau in their weight loss journey.

This is why timing matters.
Why patience matters.
Why the right sequence changes everything.

Activity: Your Energy Audit

A Moment of Honesty—Just for You

Before moving forward, take a moment to reflect:

- Where does my energy leak most right now—Physically? Emotionally? Mentally?
- Am I exhausted from effort... or from resistance?

Write it down. Not to judge yourself—but to understand where support might matter most.

Because sustainable change isn't about pushing harder.
It's about choosing the right tools at the right time.

And this book exists to help you do exactly that.

CHAPTER 15
Liposuction

The Art of Subtraction—and the Wisdom of Restraint

Liposuction is one of the most misunderstood procedures in plastic surgery—mostly because people assume it's just about "getting skinny."

It's not.

Liposuction is about **finishing**, not starting. It's about contouring...refining what you've already earned—especially when your body has done the hard work of motherhood, weight change, and recovery... yet a few stubborn areas refuse to come with you.

For the right patient, liposuction isn't a dramatic transformation. It's a quiet relief.

A smoothing.
A lightening.
A return to silhouettes that feel like *you* again.

But to do it well—and safely—requires one essential truth about the fat we are considering:

We can sculpt what's on the outside. We cannot suction what's on the inside.

The Two Types of Fat

What We Can Change—and What We Can't

There are two broad categories of fat that matter when you're planning liposuction:

1) Visceral Fat (The "Inside" Fat)

Visceral fat sits around your organs, deep inside the abdomen. It's metabolically active, and it's often what creates that firm, barrel-like belly—especially in men. If you press on the abdomen and it feels tight or solid rather than "squishy," that's often visceral fat driving the shape.

Liposuction cannot reach visceral fat.

Historically, the only reliable way to reduce it was lifestyle—nutrition, movement, sleep, stress, consistency.

More recently, medications like **GLP-1s** have changed the landscape by reducing both visceral and superficial fat for many patients. Even so, the key principle remains: visceral fat is not a liposuction target.

2) Subcutaneous Fat (The "Outside" Fat)

This is the fat just beneath the skin—the fat you can pinch. This is what we can sculpt.

And this is where liposuction shines: in the places that don't respond to effort the way they "should," even when you're doing everything right.

Where Liposuction Works Best

The "Finish Line" Zones

Liposuction is often most satisfying in areas that are small enough to refine—but meaningful enough to change how clothing fits.

Common areas include:

- Chin and neck--Say goodbye to the Turkey Gobbler
- Chest (select cases)
- Abdomen, hips, and waist ("love handles")
- Bra strap and upper back
- Inner and outer thighs
- Arms
- Underarm fold ("sleevage" / anterior axillary fold)

Some areas require extra wisdom because skin quality matters just as much as fat:

- Abdomen can be limited if the area has been repeatedly stretched (multiple pregnancies and/or Yo-Yo weight fluctuations)
- **Abdominal region** can be sequenced depending upon a patient's preference. It can be performed as a planned secondary procedure **after** a Tummy Tuck as finishing touches or as a **first step** to debulk or deflate the area in preparation for future abdominoplasty.

- **Inner thighs and arms** are notorious for looking worse if too much fat is removed but skin cannot tighten. I like to reference the "deflated bag" phenomenon that can result if over-liposuctioned.
- Like abdominoplasty, occasionally I'll recommend a deflation/debulking round of liposuction before brachioplasty (arms) or thighplasty (thighs) in order to eventually achieve a tighter contour with the skin excisional procedures. This is a situation where the patient has to agree to potentially look worse before they look better during the in-between stages.

That's why the best liposuction plans begin with the question most people don't ask:

Will your skin follow the new contour—or will it hang behind?

The Evolution of Liposuction

From "Suction" to Sculpting

Early liposuction was, frankly, aggressive—more like "put a straw in and pull." It was bloody, traumatic to tissues, and harder to control.

Modern liposuction changed everything with one major upgrade: **tumescent technique**.

We infuse a diluted fluid (typically saline or lactated Ringer's) combined with a numbing agent (lidocaine) and a blood constrictor (epinephrine) to minimize bleeding. This creates a safer environment, allows smoother removal, and dramatically improves recovery.

And because the lidocaine is diluted, the body can safely tolerate much higher total amounts in tumescent form than it could if given directly.

Safety First

Volume Limits and Why They Matter

Liposuction is not just fat removal—it's fluid balance, physiology, and careful planning.

In Tennessee, the outpatient maximum is commonly treated as **4 liters of lipoaspirate** (the total removed volume). Other states may allow 5 liters. These limits exist because higher volumes increase risks related to fluid shifts and overall physiologic stress.

In my practice, we plan with safety as the first priority—not because we're trying to be conservative, but because **a beautiful result is meaningless if it isn't safe**.

The Truth About "Types" of Liposuction

What's Real vs. What's Marketing

You'll hear endless names: Smart Lipo, Laser Lipo, Safe Lipo, Nap Time lipo... the branding can sound impressive.

The truth is simpler:

- Some devices change the *experience* of removing fat
- Some improve *precision* in certain zones
- Some help *tighten skin modestly*
  But none of them replace sound technique, seasoned experience, and honest patient selection.

The Tools I Use—and Why

VASER (Ultrasound-Assisted Liposuction)

VASER uses ultrasound energy to emulsify fat before removal. Think of it as gently loosening fat cells so they can be removed more cleanly—especially useful when we want:

- More superficial sculpting (high-definition detailing)
- Cleaner fat for transfer (because it's less mechanically traumatized)
- Precision contour work in areas where definition matters

VASER requires extra attention because the probe can heat and because technique must protect the skin at access sites. It's an excellent tool—when used thoughtfully and not casually.

Powered-Assisted Liposuction (MicroAire / PAL)

This is one of my workhorses. The handpiece vibrates the cannula, helping it glide through tissue more smoothly, with more finesse and with less aggressive force. In my opinion this makes it safer to achieve the best results and is overall less barbaric than the technique without this powered assistance.

Where it shines:

- **Chin and neck** (safer, more controlled movement)
- **Revision liposuction** (scar tissue is easier to navigate)
- **Contour corrections** (like smoothing near a C-section scar in select cases)

It's not magic.
It's **control**—and control is everything.

High-Definition Liposuction

Where Sculpture Becomes Strategy

Traditional liposuction usually stays deeper to protect blood supply to the skin and to avoid contour irregularities.

High-definition work is different. It intentionally targets more superficial layers to highlight natural anatomy—especially along the waist, abdominal lines, and the edges that create an athletic look.

For women, this is often less about the "ripped, muscular six-pack abs" and more about:

- A tightened lower waist
- A smoother transition into the hips
- A silhouette that looks clean in a bikini and effortless in clothing

This is where artistry matters—because the goal isn't to necessarily look carved.
It's to look *naturally defined.*

Skin Tightening After Liposuction

Where <u>Renuvion</u> Can Help (and Where It Can't)

After fat is removed, we're left with a honeycomb-like space under the skin and a network of fibrous bands that connect skin to deeper structures.

Renuvion uses helium plasma and radiofrequency energy to contract those fibrous bands, tightening skin by roughly **20–30%** in select patients. It has a sort of "shrink wrapping effect" on the overlying skin.

It can be a meaningful adjunct for:

- Mild to moderate laxity
- Patients who want improvement but don't want larger scars (think arms and thighs, possibly abdomen)
- Selective tightening (chin, neck, hands, labia)

But it is not a replacement for surgical excision when skin is truly excess. If someone needs a tummy tuck, arm lift, or thigh lift, no technology can "outsmart" gravity and skin biology.

A good surgeon doesn't just offer tools.
A good surgeon tells you when tools aren't enough.

Nashville Natural Notes–Practical wisdom from the consultation room

Liposuction Is About Contour, Not Weight

Liposuction is not a weight-loss procedure.

It is a sculpting tool.

The goal is not to remove as much fat as possible—it's to remove **just enough** to reveal the natural curves underneath.

Restraint creates the most beautiful results.

Who Is an Ideal Candidate?

I look at a few things right away:

1) Body Type and Distribution

Height/weight matters—but more important is what the tissue feels like. Is the fullness pinchable? Is it superficial? Is it localized?

2) Skin Quality

Age matters, but not just chronologically. Skin reflects lifestyle, genetics, sun exposure, smoking history, hydration, and weight fluctuations.

3) Expectations

If someone wants a flat, wrinkle-free abdomen but already has loose skin and stretch damage, liposuction won't deliver that outcome. That's not a moral failure. That's anatomy.

The best candidates are often women who are already doing the work—back in the gym, with consistent, stable weight—who have a few areas that simply won't cooperate.

That's where liposuction shines.

"Will the Fat Come Back?"

Liposuction removes fat cells in treated areas. Since you are only born with a defined number of fat cells, a lot of people mistakenly claim that fat *moved from one area to another.* This is just not true. If weight is gained later, fat tends to accumulate **more in untreated areas**—because those areas still have more fat cells.

But if someone gains a significant amount of weight (50–100 pounds), fat will accumulate everywhere. Liposuction is not a free pass. It's not a license to eat. It's a refinement tool—not a replacement for health.

Recovery and Results

Liposuction results are visible early—but swelling and firmness (induration) can linger. Most patients see the most meaningful refinement between **3–6 months**, with continued improvement as tissues soften.

Compression garments help:

- Reduce swelling

- Encourage smooth contouring
- Minimize fluid accumulation

If Renuvion is used, compression needs may be reduced in select cases—but good postoperative support still matters.

As for exercise: many patients can return to light activity within a week, and progress as tolerated. Soreness is usually more “bruised and tender” than truly painful.

The Real Point of Liposuction

Liposuction isn’t about chasing perfection.

It’s about removing what distracts you from the body you’ve rebuilt. It’s about alignment—between effort and outcome.

And when done well, it doesn’t make you look like someone else.

It simply helps you look like yourself again—
without the stubborn footnotes your body refused to erase on its own.

CHAPTER 16
The Tummy Truth

What Crunches Can't Fix: Your Core After Kids

"It's not just skin—it's the story of where your body's been."

For many moms, the tummy is where pregnancy leaves its loudest echoes—and its quietest wounds.

It's where joy meets biology.
Where sacrifice stretches far beyond metaphor.

And where countless women eventually whisper the same question:

"Is this really my body now?"

Many moms have colorful names for the overstretched skin that remains after pregnancy:

muffin top
mommy pooch
overhang
droopy belly skin
shelf

Or my personal favorite—**Dunlap.**

A wonderfully strange Southern phrase I learned after moving here from New Jersey, as in:

"My belly done lapped over my belt."

Humor aside, the abdominal changes after pregnancy are real.

And for many women, deeply frustrating.

Five Signs Pregnancy Changed Your Core

Many women assume their stomach simply "never went back." In reality, pregnancy often changes the **structure of the abdominal wall** in ways that exercise alone cannot correct.

If you recognize yourself in several of these signs, you may be experiencing **diastasis recti or overstretched abdominal skin**.

1. The "Mommy Pooch" That Won't Budge

Even when you lose weight or exercise regularly, the lower abdomen still pushes forward or forms a soft bulge.

This often occurs because the abdominal muscles have separated and can no longer provide strong support.

2. You Instinctively Suck In Your Stomach All Day

Many moms don't even realize they do this.

You tighten your abdomen in photos, when standing, when walking, and even while talking to people.

Over time it becomes automatic—almost like holding your breath.

3. Your Belly Button Looks Different

Pregnancy can stretch the belly button and surrounding skin.

Common changes include:

- a wider belly button
- a flattened appearance
- a "popping" or hernia-like shape

4. You Feel Weak or Unstable Through Your Core

You may notice:

- lower back fatigue
- difficulty engaging your abdominal muscles
- feeling like your center lacks strength even if the rest of your body feels strong

This happens because the muscles can no longer function as a unified support system.

5. Loose Skin That Doesn't Respond to Diet or Exercise

Even when fat decreases, the skin may remain loose or folded.

This is because stretched elastic fibers cannot fully recoil once they have been significantly overstretched.

The Important Truth

If you see yourself in these signs, it does **not** mean you didn't work hard enough after pregnancy.

It means your body adapted to create life.

And sometimes restoring that center requires more than willpower.

"Many moms believe their stomach didn't go back because they failed.
In reality, their core changed because pregnancy succeeded."

An **abdominoplasty—commonly called a tummy tuck—** done thoughtfully, safely, and in alignment with your goals—is not about vanity.
It's about *restoring your center.*

But before we talk about surgery, we need to start with a few important truths:

You cannot diet your way out of **diastasis recti.**
You cannot exercise your way out of **overstretched skin.**
You cannot positive-affirmation your way out of tissue that has been **biomechanically altered by pregnancy.**

This is not your failure.

This is your biology.

And that is where **The Tummy Truth** begins.

Before We Go Further: 3 Tummy Truths Every Mom Needs to Hear

Before we talk about muscles, skin, or surgery, there are three things every mom deserves to hear.

Because many women arrive at this chapter already quietly carrying guilt.

Let's set that down for a moment.

1. Your Body Did Exactly What It Was Designed to Do

Pregnancy asks extraordinary things of the body.

Your abdomen stretches to make room for a growing baby.
Your muscles shift.
Your skin expands.

These changes are not signs that something went wrong.

They are signs that **something miraculous happened.**

2. Not Everything Can Be Fixed With Diet and Exercise

Our culture tells women that almost everything can be solved with discipline.

Work harder.
Eat cleaner.
Exercise more.

But when connective tissue stretches apart or skin stretches beyond its elastic limits, those are structural changes.

No number of crunches can reconnect stretched fascia.

And understanding that truth should bring relief—not shame.

3. Wanting to Feel Like Yourself Again Is Not Selfish

Many moms hesitate to even consider restoring their bodies after pregnancy.

They worry it's vain.
Or indulgent.

But when a woman feels strong and confident in her body again, it changes how she moves through the world.

She stands taller.
She shows up more fully.
She models confidence for her children.

Taking care of yourself is not selfish.

Sometimes it's the first step toward becoming the version of yourself your family gets to experience every day.

Now that we've set those truths on the table, let's talk about what pregnancy actually does to the abdominal wall—and why so many moms feel like their center changed in ways they can't quite explain.

Because once you understand the anatomy, the **Tummy Truth** becomes much clearer.

What Pregnancy Really Does to the Core

The **rectus abdominis muscles**—often called the six-pack—stretch and can pull apart at the fibrous midline, creating **diastasis recti**, a literal separation of the abdominal muscles.

Your skin stretches beyond its natural limits.
Elastic fibers rupture.
The belly button widens.
Internal pressure increases.

And the muscles you rely on for posture, strength, and stability lose their ability to function as a unified team.

Many women assume they just need more exercise.

But no amount of planks or crunches can reconnect the stretched connective tissue between those muscles.

Only a surgical repair can bring them home to each other again.

This is where a tummy tuck can be life-changing—not just physically, but emotionally.

Your body didn't fail you.
It carried your children.

"The Day Emily Saw Her Core Again"

Emily, a mom of three, hadn't seen her *real* belly button in a decade.

During her exam, she cried—not from embarrassment but from relief.

"Finally," she whispered, "someone sees what I see."

Her diastasis was significant.
Her skin was overstretched.

None of it was her fault.

After surgery, she stood taller, steadier, as if her emotional core had been restored along with her physical one.

"Now my outside finally matches the woman I still feel like inside."

Sometimes we restore more than anatomy—we restore identity.

Why Skin Doesn't "Bounce Back"

Skin has limits.

Pregnancy pushes those limits.

Stretch marks form when elastic fibers snap.
Loose skin develops when the dermis expands beyond its capacity to recoil.

Creams can improve skin quality.
Exercise can tone underlying muscles.

But neither can shrink skin that has been biologically overstretched.

This is why a tummy tuck isn't cheating.

It's choosing alignment between how you *feel* inside and how you *look* outside.

The Internal Corset

One of the most important parts of a tummy tuck isn't the skin removal.

It's the restoration of the core.

During pregnancy, the abdominal muscles are pushed apart as the uterus expands.

Think of it like a corset whose laces slowly loosen over time.

When the laces are tight, the structure underneath feels supported.

When they loosen, the entire center loses stability.

During a tummy tuck, we bring those muscles back together by tightening the connective tissue in the middle.

Surgeons typically call this **rectus plication**.

I describe this as something easier to understand:

The internal corset.

The procedure doesn't change your muscles themselves.

It simply restores them to their natural position so they can function as a team again.

For many women, this is when posture improves, breathing becomes easier, and the core finally feels strong again.

"The Mom Who Finally Stopped Holding Her Breath"

Jessica admitted she had been sucking in her stomach for **twelve years**.

During her exam, I asked her to lie back and gently lift her head so her abdominal muscles engaged.

We discovered the significant separation of her diastasis recti. This is why she'd been hesitant to fully breathe for so long. She literally was holding it all in.

The moment she understood this would be tightened in an abdominoplasty, she exhaled deeply.

"That," she whispered, "is how I *used* to breathe."

After surgery, with her diastasis corrected and her abdominal muscles reoriented to proper positioned, she no longer had to suck in her stomach all day.

"This didn't just flatten my stomach—
it gave me back the breath I didn't even know I'd been holding."

Nashville Natural Notes–Practical wisdom from the consultation room

Tighter Isn't Always Better

Many patients ask for the tightest tummy possible.

But overly aggressive tightening can look unnatural and feel uncomfortable.

A great tummy tuck restores the **internal corset** and removes excess skin while preserving natural movement and contour.

The Tummy Tuck Evaluation

This part is straightforward and compassionate.
I examine:

- Skin elasticity
- Fat distribution
- Stretch marks
- Muscle separation
- C-section scarring
- Visceral vs. subcutaneous fat
- Candidacy for liposuction

And then I guide you through what's possible—not with false promises, but with precision.

Mini vs. Standard vs. Extended Tummy Tuck vs. Belt Lipectomy (Total Body Lift)

A **mini tummy tuck** removes only a small ellipse of skin below the belly button.

A **full or standard tummy tuck** allows for full tightening of the core, repositioning the belly button, and removal of the entire lower abdominal "apron." This is what we typically refer to when we discuss a Tummy Tuck or Abdominoplasty.

An **extended tummy tuck** brings the incision out wider to where the fold naturally occurs further along the side.

If the fold overlaps the sides and continues to the back —often after large weight loss—the **belt lipectomy or total body lift** is often recommended.

Most moms receive the greatest benefit from a full (standard) tummy tuck.

"The Patient Who Apologized for Her Body—Until the Day She Didn't"

Megan apologized for everything during her consult.

"Sorry... I know this is gross."
"I'm sorry you have to see this."
"I'm sorry I let myself go."

When I showed her the diastasis during her exam, she froze:

"Wait... this wasn't because I was lazy?"

Not her fault.

Not her failure.

After surgery, she never apologized again.

**"I didn't get a new stomach.
I got rid of the shame."**

The Tummy Tuck Surgery

The first step in the surgery is to release the belly button with an incision. Here, the widened, stretched-out belly button can be tightened by making the overall circumference of the opening smaller. It sits like a stalk of a flower. Think of a black-eyed Susan flower. The dark part in the middle is the belly button, and the stalk extends deep to the skin and fat. The flower is incised around the edges, and the stalk is dissected out to its base. The "stalk" of the belly button is released and awaits repositioning.

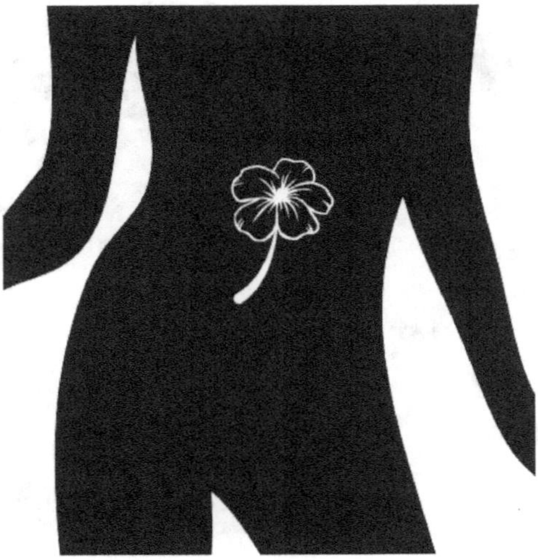

Next, a suprapubic incision that hides beneath the bikini line is made down to the muscle layer and extends in a gentle curve up toward each hip bone. This exposes a football-shaped area of skin and fat to be removed (the inch we previously pinched). The dissection continues past the belly button stalk, freeing enough tissue so it can be pulled down toward your toes, like a window shade. The rectus plication is performed next by tightening the widened fibrous band, reorienting the six-pack muscles, and then repositioning your smaller, more youthful-appearing belly button. The previously stretched-out, wrinkly football of abdominal skin and fat is punted from your body, and the incisions are closed.

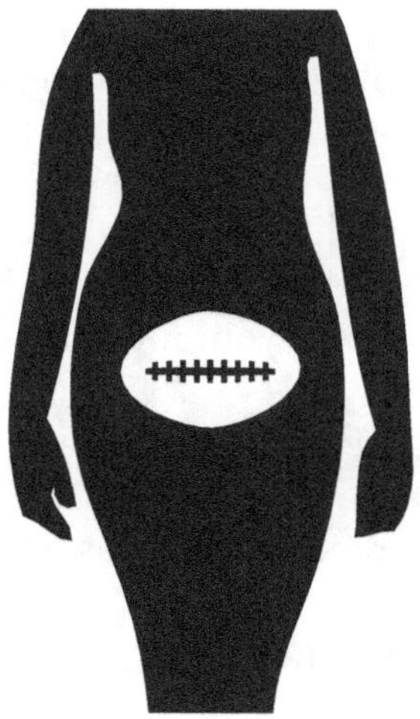

When I explain this in the office, I often use a **button-down shirt demonstration.**

The shirt button represents the belly button.

The lower seam represents the incision hidden beneath underwear.

I dissect up under the shirt toward the rib cage, perform the "internal corset" of the rectus plication, pull the shirt down, and any bunched-up excess is excised and thrown into the trash.

The belly button is repositioned in a more youthful and vertical position, and the lower incision is closed.

Voilà! A smoother, flatter, younger tummy!

How the Surgery Works — In Clear, Human Terms

Here's what happens:

- The belly button is released and refined
- The lower incision is placed low for concealment
- The abdominal flap is lifted
- The midline is repaired—your internal corset
- Excess skin is removed
- The belly button is rebuilt and repositioned
- Liposuction is added if needed
- Everything is closed with precision

The result?
A flatter silhouette, a smoother front profile, and a stronger physical center.

What a Great Tummy Tuck Should <u>Never</u> Do

A tummy tuck, when done thoughtfully and safely, can be transformative.

But like any powerful procedure, **how it's done matters**.

Here are a few things a well-performed tummy tuck should **<u>never</u>** do.

1. It Should <u>Never</u> Look "Pulled" or Artificial

A good tummy tuck restores your natural abdominal contour.

It should not look overly tight, flattened like a board, or unnatural when you move.

The goal is **balance and harmony**, not an artificially stretched appearance.

2. It Should <u>Never</u> Leave the Belly Button Looking Fake

One of the most common signs of poor technique is an unnatural belly button.

It may appear:

- perfectly round
- overly large
- placed too high
- surrounded by visible scarring

A natural belly button should look **subtle, vertical, and unnoticeable**.

In great surgery, most people won't even realize you had one.

3. It Should Never Be Placed Too High

A properly designed tummy tuck incision sits **low enough to be hidden in underwear or a swimsuit**.

If the scar is placed too high, patients may struggle to conceal it in normal clothing.

Careful planning and experience are critical to getting this right.

4. It Should Never Compromise Safety for Aggressiveness

Sometimes patients request extremely tight results.

But an ethical surgeon balances aesthetics with **circulation, healing, and long-term safety**.

Too much tension on the skin can increase complications and delay healing.

The best results come from **precision, not force**.

5. It Should Never Make You Feel Ashamed of Your Body

A good consultation should feel respectful and educational.

You should never feel judged, rushed, or pressured into surgery.

The right surgeon helps you understand your options and supports you in making the decision that's best for you.

The Real Goal

A beautiful tummy tuck doesn't announce itself.

It simply restores the natural shape your body once had.

When done well, people don't say:

"Nice surgery."

They say:

"You look amazing."

Great surgery doesn't create a new body.
It restores the one that pregnancy changed.

A Word on Massive Weight Loss Patients

Patients who have lost **50 pounds or more** may require a circumferential approach called a **belt lipectomy or total body lift**.

This removes excess skin around the abdomen and back, often improving the outer thighs and buttocks as well.

The goal is to tighten the body while preserving comfort and natural movement.

"The Grocery Store Streaker"

One of my patients had lost a significant amount of weight and underwent a circumferential belt lipectomy along with breast surgery. Two weeks later—feeling proud, a little stir-crazy, and ready to reclaim normal life—she decided to stop by the grocery store on her way to a postoperative visit.

She wore loose sweatpants with a drawstring waistband.

Unfortunately, somewhere between the produce section and checkout, that drawstring quietly surrendered.

Because the scars from surgery were still numb, she didn't feel a thing.

Not the gradual loosening.

Not the slipping fabric.

Nothing.

Until suddenly she felt a cool breeze across her thighs.

She looked down.

Her sweatpants were around her ankles.

In the middle of the grocery store.

She pulled them up as quickly as a two-week postoperative patient reasonably can, apologized to the startled clerk, and shuffled out of the store as fast as dignity—and her healing incisions—would allow.

When she told me the story at her follow-up appointment, she was laughing so hard she nearly slid off the exam table.

Her new nickname for herself?

"The grocery store streaker."

What struck me most was her attitude. Instead of embarrassment, she felt pride. Losing that much weight and reclaiming her body had been a huge accomplishment.

And if there was a lesson in the whole experience, she said, it was this:

After years of never needing one...it was finally time to start wearing a belt again.

Recovery — Truth, Compassion, and Reassurance

The first few days tend to be the hardest.

Walking helps.
Pain medication helps.
Time helps.

And support from others helps most of all.

This is not the time for hustle.

It's the time for stillness, patience, and letting others care for you for once.

Your scar will fade.
Your numbness will resolve.
Your core will strengthen.
Your confidence will rise.

And your results—done right, cared for properly—can last for years.

Beware –The Southern Mom's Dilemma

Sarah struggled with what she described for me as the Southern Mom's Dilemma about considering plastic surgery (although I've seen this in varied forms in moms from all parts of the country):

After children, a mom experiences diastasis recti and stretched out skin in her midsection. The patient feels that it is a medical issue and not just cosmetic vanity (which I agree with). So, because the diastasis recti is an after-effect of pregnancy, it's a medical issue. Medical issues should be covered by insurance→ If it's not covered by insurance, it's cosmetic→

If it's purely cosmetic, it's vanity→If it's vanity→ it's a Sin because it takes away money and resources from the family. Therefore, wanting to fix effects of pregnancy, i.e. the diathesis recti, the mom pooch, is sinful.

While I understand and can empathize with these moms, I'm of the opinion that God wants us to be our best and, if there is an after-effect of pregnancy that we can fix and don't, I'll counter that that could be considered sinful.

If a mom avoids taking her children to the pool because she is concerned about people staring at her overhanging mom pooch, that is more sinful than focusing a bit on herself. In my mind, God and the bible determine what is sinful, certainly not some insurance company.

I've often wondered about my part in all this as I've traveled my own faith journey. I've realized that God gave me specials skills and ability to connect with patients to fix those things for moms who are impacted by their body after childbirth. I rely on God to guide me, steer me and be with me as I use these skills to make a mom's life (and her family's life) better.

I believe God wants each of us to live life to the fullest and become our best selves. If the after-effects of pregnancy prevent a mom from returning to her true self, uncovering her authentic self, or stepping fully into her confident self, that should be avoided or fixed if possible. A confident mom teaches her children confidence and that Ripple effect is unmatched. That resource is priceless.

"The Woman Who Finally Wore the Dress She Saved for Someday"

Melissa had kept a navy blue wrap dress in her closet for eight years.

She always said she would wear it "someday."

After her tummy tuck, she walked into my office wearing it.

"Someday," she said, "arrived today."

"This wasn't about looking skinny.
It was about feeling like *me* again."

The Tummy Truth in 30 Seconds

If you remember nothing else from this chapter, remember this:

Pregnancy changes the body in real structural ways.

Diastasis recti is not a failure of discipline.

Wanting your body to feel strong again is not vanity.

A well-performed tummy tuck restores more than appearance.

And the real goal is not perfection.

It's feeling at home in your body again.

Your body didn't fail you...it carried your children.

Chapter Exercise

Release What You've Been Holding In

For many moms, the stomach isn't just where pregnancy changed the body.

It's also where years of tension and self-criticism quietly live.

Try this simple exercise.

Place one hand over your abdomen.

Take a slow breath in through your nose.

Allow your stomach to expand naturally.

Then exhale slowly.

Many women notice something surprising:

They've been holding their stomach in for years.

Now write the answer to this question:

"For years, I've been holding in..."

Be honest.

It might be:

- embarrassment
- frustration
- disappointment
- anger at your body
- exhaustion from trying to "fix" something that wasn't your fault

Write whatever comes up.

Then write one more sentence:

"What I want to feel in my body again is..."

Strength.
Ease.
Freedom.
Confidence.

There is no right answer.

One Final Question

Ask yourself this gently:

"If my body could support me again instead of something I constantly fight, how would my life feel different?"

Write the answer.

You may be surprised how emotional this becomes.

Because restoring your center is rarely just about your abdomen.

Sometimes it's simply about finally exhaling after years of holding it all in.

Closing Reflection

Your abdomen carried life.

It stretched.
It adapted.
It sacrificed.

And if part of your journey now includes restoring that center, that choice doesn't erase the past.

It honors it.

Because the truth has been there all along:

Your body didn't fail you.
It carried your children.

CHAPTER 17
The Breast Story

Reclaiming the Feminine: The Post-Baby Breast Journey

"You fed life from your body—it's okay to want to feel balanced again."

Breasts tell a story long before a woman ever speaks a word.

They tell the story of pregnancy, nursing, sleepless nights, hormones that rose and crashed like waves, and the tug-of-war between nurturing others and remembering yourself. They tell the story of a mother's generosity—and sometimes, the physical cost of it.

I meet women every week who sit down in my consultation room, take a breath that sounds more like an apology, and whisper:

"I don't recognize them anymore."
or
"I didn't love them before kids, and now they're... gone."
or simply
"Can you help?"

And the truth is: *Yes. We can.*

Not because you're "vain."
Not because you're "fixing" something broken.
But because you deserve to feel at home in your body again.

Breast surgery—augmentation, lift, reduction, or refinement—is not about becoming someone new.
It's about **returning** to yourself... or discovering the version of you that motherhood muted.

What Really Happens to Breasts After Baby

Pregnancy reshapes the breasts in ways diet and exercise can't undo.
Volume expands with milk production.
Skin stretches beyond its limits.
The nipple-areola complex widens.
Breastfeeding adds pulling, tugging, tension, and swelling.

Then, almost overnight, everything **deflates**.

The fullness you once had on top becomes hollow.
The lower pole descends.
Elasticity gives way to gravity.
Symmetry disappears.
Your reflection feels foreign.

None of this is your fault.
None of it is failure.
All of it is biology.

And all of it is *fixable*.

Patient Story — "Rolling Them Into My Bra"

She walked in with a brave smile—the kind moms wear when they're trying not to fall apart.

"I used to have small breasts," she said. "Not great, but mine."
She nursed all three of her kids, right up until baby number three was ten months.

"And now?" I asked gently.

Her face crumpled.

"They're... worse. The little I had is gone. I have to roll them into my bra. Please tell me I'm not stuck like this."

When I told her the truth—that what she was experiencing was normal, common, and absolutely correctable—she exhaled so deeply it was as if she'd been holding that breath for years.

"I just wanted to feel like myself again. Thank you for seeing me."

The Two Questions That Shape Everything

When we start discussing options, I always ask:

1. **Do you desire fullness—or do you desire to be perky?**
2. **What would feeling confident again actually look like for you?**

Some women want to restore what they had.
Some want the volume they never got to experience.
Some want less volume, but more balance.

Some want symmetry.
Some want simplicity—breasts that fit a bra without a fight.

And some don't know what they want yet—they just know what they *don't* want:

- the emptiness
- the droop
- the mismatch
- the constant adjusting
- the shame

Breast surgery is a conversation long before it's an operation.

"The Locker Room Confession"

Danielle had been embarrassed about her chest since middle school. Pregnancy only made the contrast between her and "everyone else" feel louder.

She walked into my office folded into herself—arms across her chest, shoulders hunched, voice barely above a whisper.

"When I look in the mirror, I feel like a 13 year old boy."

But when she tried on implants during our sizing session—when she saw possibility reflected back at her—something shifted.

Her posture lifted.
Her eyes softened.
Her voice warmed.

After surgery, she walked in glowing.

"I can't stop looking at myself. I finally feel feminine. I finally feel... right."

Timing Matters — But Not as Much as You Think

Ideally, we perform breast procedures when:

- You're done breastfeeding (3–6 months after weaning)
- Your breasts have stabilized
- Your weight is close to normal
- You're not planning another pregnancy soon

But life isn't always linear.

Unexpected pregnancies happen.
Bodies shift.
Plans change.

With modern surgical techniques, many women still breastfeed after lifts or augmentations—and enjoy stable results.

We talk through all this.
No pressure.
No pushing.
Just clarity.

Let's Talk About the Reality of Choice

There is no "one right option."
There is only the right option **for you**.

Breast augmentation

For the mom who says:

- "They disappeared."
- "I just want to feel feminine again."
- "I want my cleavage back."

Breast lift (mastopexy)

For the mom who says:

- "They're too low, even if I fill them."
- "My nipples point down."
- "I want perkiness—not size."

Lift + implant

For the mom who says:

- "I want both fullness and elevation."
- "I want to look like me—only better."
- "I don't want the Snoopy look."

Breast reduction

For the mom who says:

- "I have back pain."
- "I can't exercise."
- "I want freedom."

Areola or nipple refinement

For the mom who says:

- "They look stretched."
- "They look uneven."
- "They bother me in bras or swimsuits."

Every option is valid.
Every desire is legitimate.
Every woman deserves the shape that matches her spirit.

"The Anniversary Surprise"

Raquel wanted breast surgery as a gift for her twelfth anniversary--for her husband, she said.

But the truth unfolded afterward:
she did it for *both* of them.

"I just want to feel pretty again," she said softly.
"I want my husband to see the woman he fell in love with."

After surgery, she laughed when I asked how he was handling the change:

"Oh, I haven't let him touch them yet!
He's like a starved cheetah staring at antelopes.
And honestly? I'm loving every minute of it."

At her next visit:
"He's so proud of me...and you, too Doc! And so am I. I'm so, so proud of myself."

Confidence is attractive.
Comfortable, reclaimed confidence even more so.

Activity: "Confidence, for me, looks like..."

Write this sentence at the top of a page.

Complete it without editing, apologizing, or shrinking.

Let your truth speak first.

You're not choosing breasts—you're choosing how you want to *feel* in your body for the next decade.

CHAPTER 18

Fuller, Not Fake: Breast Augmentation That Looks Like You—Only Better

For many moms, the most surprising change after childbirth isn't in their belly—
it's in their breasts.

The fullness that once gave shape to a blouse or swimsuit quietly disappears.
Cleavage softens, volume drops, and the upper pole deflates.
Women describe this moment in a hundred different ways, but the meaning is always the same:

Something changed...
and it hasn't come back.

But here's the truth most moms never hear:

You were able to feed life from your body.
It's okay to want to feel balanced again.

Breast augmentation isn't about being "done."
It isn't about being flashy.
It's about restoring harmony—inside and out.

It's about reclaiming the curve that motherhood softened,
and choosing a version of yourself that feels aligned with who you are now.

And in my practice, that philosophy has a name:

Nashville Natural™ — Where Beauty Whispers, Not Shouts

When I talk to moms about augmentation, most say something like:

"I don't want to look fake—I want to look like me... just perky."

Or:

"I want to look amazing on date nights,
but I don't want to make a scene at preschool pickup."

That's why our guiding aesthetic is what I call **Nashville Natural**:

- Polished, not obvious
- Elegant, not exaggerated
- Confidence that blends in all day
- Curves you can amplify at night

Nashville Natural™ is the aesthetic sweet spot where art, anatomy, and authenticity meet.
It's the look that makes people lean in and wonder:

- **"Did she... or didn't she?"**
- It's enhancement without announcement—
a result that elevates your silhouette without overpowering it.

You look incredible—
but no one quite knows why.

That's Nashville Natural.

"Mom With Those... Not THOSE."

There's a moment in consult when I'll see a patient struggling to enunciate her desired shape and size. There is a concern between wanting enhancement and fearing the over-obvious result where judgment can be an unwelcomed consequence.

I like to confer with my patients to understand their vision. I'll clarify by asking them, "When you're at the ballfield with your kids, you'll want to be referred to as the "mom with those (referring to her children) and not the mom with THOSE (meaning her overly large implants), right?" Every mom laughs.

Because every mom understands exactly what that means. And that is NOT Nashville Natural.

Breast augmentation should fit your:

- lifestyle
- family season
- wardrobe
- personality
- identity

It should make you feel beautiful—
not make you feel like you're performing.

Nashville Natural Notes-Practical wisdom from the consultation room

Breasts Should Match the Body

Implants that overwhelm the body rarely look natural.

The best breast surgery respects the patient's height, frame, and proportions.

The goal isn't necessarily "bigger."

The goal is **balanced**.

"The Day She Dared to Look in the Mirror"

Anna hadn't worn a V-neck since her second child was born.

She told me:

"It feels like my chest collapsed."

During sizing, when she saw herself in the mirror with the implant samples in place, she froze.
Then her eyes filled with tears.

"This looks like... me.
The me I remember."

Two months after surgery, she came in wearing the softest smile and a wrap dress she'd been saving for years.

"I'm not hiding anymore," she said.
"Not my body. Not my joy."

This isn't vanity.
This is restoration.

Where Artistry Meets Anatomy:

The Music City Plastic Surgery 5-Star Sizing System™ & 6-String Assessment™

Breast augmentation is deeply visual. You don't get Nashville Natural results by guesswork. It requires conversation, intuition, anatomy, and mathematical harmony.

My **5-Star Sizing System**™ helps translate your vision into surgical reality.

I joke that I like to get "inside" my patient's head. In reality, breast augmentation surgery—and sizing in particular—is such a visual exchange. There are many variables that need to be elucidated from the patient's perspective in order to get the perfect result.

That's why I created two complementary tools:

The 5-Star Sizing System™, which reveals what you *see* for yourself...
and
The 6-String Assessment™, which reveals what your *body* is designed for.

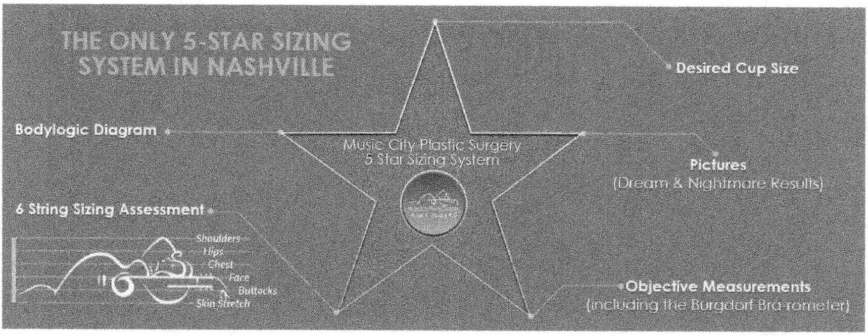

One is your voice.
The other is your instrument.

Together, they allow us to create a result that feels inevitable—
as if your body had been waiting for this all along.

1. ☆ Bodylogic Diagram

I'll show you a set of simple side-view sketches that progress from subtle to fuller projection. They're not technical—just gentle visuals to help you sense what feels right.

Most moms hover between two drawings. That hesitation isn't confusion; it's clarity emerging. And you don't need to overthink it. These sketches simply elucidate your preferences for both of us.

Often, the drawing you select aligns with the cup size you believe you want.
But occasionally, there's a mismatch—

a reminder that bra sizing is an inconsistent fashion language at best... and many moms have never pictured themselves beyond the size they've lived in for years.

More than once, a patient has said,
"*I don't even know what cup size I want.*
I can't imagine what a ___ cup would look like on me."

That's perfectly normal.
These sketches help you choose not by a letter—
but by the shape and confidence you want to step into.

2. ☆Desired Cup Size

Not a promise.
A direction.
A shared language for your goals and a jumping off point to start the conversation.

*A quick side note: Many women use their friend's experience with an augmentation as a reference point. I hear "My friend had 350cc, and I think that would be perfect for me too." While this can also be that entry door into the conversation, I caution against strong adherence to this exact size. No two women are the same. Aside from starting cup size, each woman is likely to have different life experiences that will impact her. From hereditary influences, to number of pregnancies, with amount of weight gained/lost, time spent breast feeding, if at all, to other life choices like diet, smoking, sun exposure, to inherent chest skin integrity, etc. The variables are innumerable. While I am thankful for the friend's positive experience with plastic surgery, I am strict in my belief of treating each patient individually. There is no cookie cutter answer in my practice.

3. ☆Dream Photos & Nightmare Photos

Dream Photos: Pictures of "your perfect look"—cleavage, fullness, overall vibe.

Nightmare Photos: Just as important. What you absolutely *don't* want. This protects your final result from drifting too large/ too artificial or too small leading to underwhelm/disappointment.

Another element for Visual clarity of YOUR desired look.

4. ☆Objective Measurements

Chest wall dimensions
Tissue elasticity
Breast base width
Nipple position
Rib arc and curvature
Measurements to determine symmetry vs asymmetry

This is where **science meets soul**—
the exact place Nashville Natural™ lives.

5. ☆The 6 String Sizing Assessment- a combination of Objective & Subjective Factors.

The 6-String Assessment™

Because no woman is one-dimensional. Think of your body as an instrument—
six strings that must be tuned to create harmony.

During your "sizing session" of trying on implant samples, I evaluate six parameters of your anatomy:

1. **Shoulders**
2. **Chest / Ribcage Anatomy**
3. **Hips**
4. **Backside / Posterior Curve**
5. **Skin Stretch & Elasticity**
6. **Face** (this is often the subtle "tell" that lets me know when we've reached that "perfect size").

When these six elements align, the result is simply breathtaking—natural, proportionate, unmistakably *you.*

When all six strings resonate—shoulders, chest, hips, backside, skin, and even your facial expression—something extraordinary happens: your anatomy tells me, without a word, when we've found the size that feels like *home.*

And that is where the real artistry begins.

I use what I call the Goldilocks approach during the sizing session. We try on *too small*, *just right*, and *intentionally too large*—so you can clearly see the full spectrum and never walk away wondering, *"Should I have gone bigger?"* This takes the pressure off you to guess or overthink; your eyes and intuition will tell us everything we need to know.

Unlike some surgeons, I don't expect my patients to choose their implant size on their own. I absolutely value your vision and your preference—but you're not expected to understand tissue behavior, breast asymmetries, or the subtle structural differences that make one size look perfect and another look forced. Every breast has its own history, its own limitations, its own possibilities.

We will evaluate the choices in the mirror together. We will look with you facing forward and looking at your projection from the side. I will take all the factors within the 6-String Assessment into consideration.

As you face the mirror, we will assess how each size fits within your frame of chest, shoulders, hips. Turning sideways, we will assess your projection up top and relate it in your proportion with your backside. Like a patient recently told me, "*Don't make me look like the Letter P*", referring to having overly large implants with a smaller backside.

And finally, I examine your face. There's always a point during this sizing session where I can tell by the look upon your face that we've hit the right size. There's a bit of a twinkle in the eye, a bit of a sigh of relaxation, a sort of "this feels right" look that often the patient doesn't even recognize herself. But I see it and I make sure it's brought to life in the operating room.

So, we do this together: your desires, my expertise.

With your guidance—not your burden—I translate the story your body has lived into the shape you want to step into. That partnership is the art behind the science of breast surgery.

Dress Them Up, Blend Them In

Breast augmentation has never truly been about size.
It's about range.
It's about having a body that moves with you—
not one that announces itself before you do.

Breast augmentation is about a body that adapts to you—
quietly confident in the daylight,
effortlessly captivating when the lights are low.

Most moms want this exact harmony:

In the everyday rhythms—carpool lines, grocery aisles, school bleachers—
your breasts feel balanced, comfortable, natural...
a kind of beauty no one can quite put their finger on.

But when evening comes—dinner with your spouse, date nights, anniversaries—
you can "dress them up":
a touch more curve, a sweep of cleavage,
a silhouette that whispers confidence without ever shouting for attention.

This is why the sizing matters.
Why precision matters.
Why artistry and restraint matter.

Because you should never have to choose between elegance and feeling beautiful.

With the right approach, you get both—
a look that blends in when you want it to...
and lights up a room when you're ready.

Nashville Natural™ means:

she looks incredible...
but no one can quite tell why.

Not "done."
Not obvious.
Just beautifully *her.*

It's breast augmentation in harmony—
artistry tuned so well that people wonder:
"Did she... or didn't she?"

That is the signature of proportion.
That is the hallmark of mastery.
That is Nashville Natural™.

"The Mom Who Wanted to Look Good in T-Shirts—Not Just Lingerie"

Caroline told me during her consult:
"I don't want to look 'done.' I just want to look good in a plain white T-shirt."

That became our guiding North Star.

At her 6-week visit, she walked in wearing exactly that—
a fitted white tee and jeans.
She turned to the mirror, smiled, and said:

"*This is who I was always meant to be.*"

Not louder.
Not showy.
Just right.

"Elegance isn't created by going bigger.
It's created by going truer."

A breast that blends in when you wish
and lights up the room when you choose
is the very definition of Nashville Natural™.

What Breast Augmentation Truly Offers Moms

- Not attention — but alignment
- Not exaggeration — but elegance
- Not a spectacle — but a homecoming

It gives you the chance to see yourself again—
not the version motherhood stretched thin,
but the version you remember...
and sometimes the version you always hoped one day to meet.

And that's the heart of it:
breast augmentation isn't about becoming someone else—
it's about reclaiming the spectrum of confidence that already belongs to you.

But before any of that can happen—
before the T-shirt fits just right
or the evening gown makes your reflection catch your breath—
you deserve clarity.

You deserve truth.
And that begins with the question every mother eventually asks, whether boldly or softly:

"Are breast implants safe?"

**"Before beauty, before sizing, before artistry—
every woman deserves certainty."**

Are Breast Implants Safe?

The Question Every Mom Deserves to Ask—Out Loud

Yes.
They are.

Earlier generations of implants had issues—too many unknowns, too many questions without clear answers.
So the industry paused. Rethought. Reformulated.

After years of research and testing, silicone gel implants returned to the market stronger, safer, more stable, and far less likely to ripple or rupture. The newer "form-stable" gels—what most people call *gummy bears*—are even more reliable, holding their shape the way a good memory foam cushion does: giving when needed, supporting when it counts.

No scientific study has ever established a cause-and-effect link between implants and autoimmune disease.

Are there risks?
Of course—there are with every surgical procedure.

But modern implants are safe, refined, regulated, and trusted by millions of women who simply wanted to feel like themselves again.

The Breast Augmentation Procedure

A Blend of Precision and Poise

Breast augmentation is quick—usually 35–45 minutes—
but the planning is meticulous.

Before the implant ever enters your body, we make several decisions together:

Creating the Pocket

Where the Implant Will Live

Think of the "pocket" as the seat your implant sits in.
It can be placed:

• **Subglandular (above the muscle)** — natural breast tissue over muscle
• **Submuscular (beneath the muscle)** — my go-to
• **Dual plane (part muscle, part tissue)** — especially for moms wanting upper-pole fullness without a full lift

Most of my Mommy Makeover patients benefit beautifully from the **submuscular or dual-plane** approach.
These positions:

- disguise the upper edge of the implant
- look more natural
- reduce rippling
- improve mammogram accuracy
- age gracefully

A pocket that's too aggressively dissected can shift or rotate, giving the dreaded "side boob" that creeps toward your armpit.
A carefully sculpted pocket keeps the implant centered, stable, and elegant.

Incision Location: The Hidden Entry Point

Your incision is typically placed in the **inframammary fold**—the natural crease where your breast meets your chest wall.

It's discreet. Precise.
And fades quickly.

Could we go through the armpit or around the nipple?
Technically yes, but it often compromises precision or increases risk.

My priority is results that are safe, beautiful, and durable.

Love the Cleavage, Hate the Sleevage—An accessory procedure that can make all the difference.

One area that is often inquired about when discussing breasts involve the area that gets pushed up and more pronounced when wearing a bra. This "sleevage" is frustrating for many women, especially in thin individuals. Often, this can be addressed by bringing the breast in a more projecting position with an implant. But, for those with a little extra fatty tissue here, a quick bit of liposuction can eliminate this bulge of the "sleevage".

Waking Up to Your New Reflection

When you first wake from surgery, your breasts may sit higher than expected—almost like they're standing at attention.

Don't panic.

Over the next **2–4 weeks**, they soften, settle, and find their natural, Nashville-Natural position.

Nearly every woman has a moment during healing where she thinks:

"Are they too big?"
followed later by
"Are they too small?"

That emotional roller coaster is part of the journey.
Give your body time to heal and your eyes time to adjust.

Almost always, the final verdict becomes:

"They're perfect."

After the Surgery

Your Recovery, Simplified

You'll go home the same day, in a soft sports bra and with a chest that feels tight, full, and a bit sore—like the day after a chest workout magnified by 10.

Here's the rhythm of recovery:

• **Days 1–2:** Rest, Netflix, hydration, gentle walking
• **Day 2–3:** Showering is allowed
• **Day 3:** Begin gentle arm stretches to help the implants settle
• **Week 1:** I'll see you to check healing & teach you implant-specific massage
• **Weeks 2–6:** No heavy lifting, intense workouts, or straining
• **Weeks 6+:** You begin to feel truly "normal" again as all activities are allowed now

I like performing surgery Thursday or Friday so you can be back to work and life on Monday (in most cases).

Watching Confidence Bloom

Moments I'll Never Forget

Danielle

When Danielle first came in, she folded into herself like she wished she could disappear.
She apologized for her chest as if it were a flaw in her character, not her anatomy.

After surgery?

She walked in with light in her eyes.
Shoulders back.
Voice steady.
She said: *"I can't stop looking at myself. I finally feel like a woman."*

I almost didn't recognize her—
not because her body changed,
but because **her confidence exploded**.

Maintaining Your Results

What Time, Gravity & Life Can Influence

Your implants are stable—
but **your tissue** is alive, changing, aging, stretching.

Your long-term results depend on:

- Weight stability
- Pregnancy/breastfeeding
- Your skin's elasticity (impacted by genetic and life-decision factors)
- Implant size (bigger = more strain over time)

Small, tasteful implants often age best—another reason the Nashville Natural philosophy holds up beautifully over the years.

Possible Complications

Rare, but Worth Understanding

All safe surgeries still carry risks.
Here's what we look out for:

Capsular Contracture

Your body forms a soft scar capsule around the implant—normal.
But if it tightens too much, the breast may feel firm or look distorted.

Rupture

With saline, it's obvious—like a deflated balloon.
With gel, it's usually silent due to the stable shape of modern implants. A significant force would typically be required for a rupture of silicone gel implants.

Rippling

More common in very thin patients with saline implants.
Almost nonexistent with form-stable gels.

These issues are *uncommon*, and when they do occur,
we're very experienced at addressing them.

Mammograms & Implants

Yes—You Still Get Them

You'll continue your routine mammogram schedule.

Your tech will use the **Eklund view**, which gently shifts the implant back and pulls the natural breast tissue forward.
It might sound technical, but it's really a simple adjustment.

God Bless America and God Bless Jennifer

You've earlier learned about the anniversary surprise of Raquel's breast augmentation. But I want to introduce you to Jennifer, a military wife, who approached me with an idea that made me even more proud to be an American than I already was.

She told me of her husband's deployment and her idea of a "Welcome Home Breast Augmentation Surprise." I was honored to be a part of this. I was all in. I'm a big fan of and big believer in thanking anyone in the military for their service, but this takes it to a whole other level.

When he accompanied Jennifer to one of her follow-up appointments, I got the chance to shake his hand and offer my thanks for what he did for our country. When I asked him about the surprise his wife orchestrated, all he could say was "The sacrifice was well worth it!" Haha!

God Bless America!

The Heart of It All

Breast augmentation—done thoughtfully, conservatively, and artistically—isn't vain.

It's liberating.

It's the quiet confidence in a T-shirt.
It's the joy of dressing up and feeling magnetic again.
It's your reflection matching the woman you've always been on the inside.

That is the Nashville Natural promise:
Whisper, don't shout.
Elegance first.
Confidence always.

CHAPTER 19

Lifting Without Overdoing: Breast Lifts that Reshape Without Shocking Your Reflection

From Nourishment to Renewal

There is a quiet poetry in the way a mother's breasts change over time.

They swell with purpose.
They soften with sacrifice.
They nourish, sustain, and give—
often without ever being replenished.

Many women tell me, almost in a whisper:

"I gave life through my body... but I lost parts of myself along the way."

A breast lift is not about vanity.
It is about alignment—bringing your outer shape back into resonance with the woman you know yourself to be. Many of my Mommy Makeover patients tell me that they want to restore their breasts to their pre-children form.

This chapter is not an invitation to become someone new.
It is an invitation to come home.

Your Breasts After Baby

What Changed—and Why It Matters

Pregnancy and breastfeeding place extraordinary demands on the breasts.

Hormonal swelling expands tissue.
Milk production stretches the skin envelope.
Breastfeeding traction strains the internal support system.
And when weaning is complete, the breasts often deflate more than recovers and loses their elasticity—their lift. They become droopy and just flop on the chest.

Of all the sacrifices moms make for their kids, sagging breasts are often one of the most visible.

Common changes include:

- Loss of upper-pole (upper-breast) fullness
- Downward migration of the breast mound
- Nipples that no longer face forward
- Skin laxity and tissue thinning
- Increasing asymmetry between sides

These changes are normal.
But they are rarely welcome.

Exercise, posture, skincare, and supportive bras all contribute to wellness—but they cannot correct structural changes caused by pregnancy physiology.

That is where surgery becomes a tool.
Not for transformation—but for restoration.

A breast lift—medically called a mastopexy—repositions the breast mound to a more youthful, natural location, reshapes the tissue, and re-centers the nipple so the breast sits comfortably on the chest again.

Some moms have always wanted larger breasts; some just want them back up in their original position; some want their nipples not to point to the floor. Some women actually loved the fullness, the increased cleavage, of their breasts while they were pregnant and want them to look like that now.

How I Assess Breast Lift Readiness

The Questions Behind the Consultation.

During your consult, I'm listening for alignment and I'll ask questions like:

- When you think about your breasts before kids—what do you miss most?
- Was it the size... or where they sat on your chest?
- Do you like your volume, but not your position?
- Are your nipples facing forward—or South?

- What do you find yourself adjusting during the day? Bras? Straps? Posture? Clothing?

These answers guide everything.

One of our goals for you is to have congruent breasts that have a natural appearance and shape.

A Word of Caution:

Often, women try to avoid a breast lift surgery and only want to use an implant in attempts to achieve a full lift. If they truly need a lift, this is usually a poor decision. It could lead to using way too large of an implant resulting in a heavy-set appearance or, if using an appropriate size implant for her chest wall, can result in a shape known as "Snoopy dog deformity."

Without the lift, there is a disconnect between the fullness created by the implant and the rest of the drooping breast—the nipple is the dog's nose pointing down. By lifting the breast tissue up on top of an implant, we can achieve a nicer cascade to the breast that has a natural-looking effect.

Lift Alone or Lift with Augmentation?

A Structural Decision—Not a Trend

A lift restores position.
It does not always restore fullness.

Pregnancy often flattens the upper portion of the breast. In these cases, adding a modest implant can restore balance—not size for size's sake, but harmony between structure and volume.

We can discuss the advantages of coupling the lift with an

augmentation, not just for size but for symmetry, uniformity, and the overall look of the breasts when we are done. Doing a breast lift usually involves removing some tissue from the lower aspect of the breast. Augmentation with a breast implant compensates for these losses of volume and rounds out the result nicely. Using my advanced surgical techniques, I can perform both procedures at the same time, very safely.

This is why many Mommy Makeover patients choose a lift with augmentation:
not to be bigger, but to be proportionate.

As discussed in the Breast Augmentation chapter, Nashville Natural™ results depend on restraint—never using volume to compensate for structure.

Internal Bra? Aka Galaflex

Another element to consider with breast lift is an additional support substance known as Galaflex or the "Internal Bra" as we like to call it at Music City Plastic Surgery. GalaFlex is a dissolvable mesh made from a suture-like material that helps to support the breasts from within, acting as a natural scaffolding to elevate the bust. It can be used during breast augmentation, breast lift, breast reduction, or breast revision to enhance results, defy aesthetic complications, and create more lasting, positive changes.

The mesh gradually disintegrates over the course of several years, during which time the body replaces the Internal Bra with its own collagen. The lower chest thus develops five to ten times the strength of natural breast tissue, allowing the breasts to better resist gravity, weight fluctuations, and the aging process.

What Are the Benefits of GalaFlex?

As a dissolvable scaffold to elevate and support the breasts, GalaFlex has many advantages. It acts like a built-in hammock, cradling the breasts over the course of several years as the patient's body regenerates new collagen to replace this internal bra. The GalaFlex mesh is absorbed, leaving behind breast tissue that is approximately five times more robust.

Additional benefits of the GalaFlex internal bra:

- Reduces stress on the lower breast skin, which has proven to be inherently unreliable in maintaining support of the breast substance
- Provides additional breast implant support, allowing for expanded options of implant size selection.
- Long-lasting structural improvement
- Helps maintain cleavage by cradling the lower hemisphere of the breast as a built-in bra
- Reduces the need for revision surgeries
- Helps create a rounder, more attractive breast shape
- Prevents complications such as bottoming out or lateral displacement of an implant
- Controls the pocket size when downsizing or exchanging implants
- Boosts collagen production

Who is a candidate for Galaflex?

Galaflex has been a game changer in my practice over the last dozen or so years. I offer it in nearly every breast lift case, especially those moms who have multiple children or who have had frequent weight fluctuations. I often refer to the "overstretched rubber band phenomenon" of the lower breast skin that occurs with the expansion during pregnancy/ breastfeeding and the subsequent deflation aftermath once weaned. I all but mandate this in massive weight loss patience or those with greater than three children. I consider it a bit of an insurance policy to maintain the results and achieve better longevity in the breast shape. I often tell my patients that I love to operate... but rather than do their breast lift several times in a short time span because results were not maintained, I would rather operate on them once the right way... and then all of their friends too because they were so pleased with the results.

"I Didn't Want Bigger—Just Back."

Melissa sat quietly and finally said:

"I don't need more. I just want them where they used to be."

After her lift, she came in wearing a fitted sweater and laughed softly.

"I forgot what it felt like not to adjust myself all day."

Not bigger.
Not different.
Just hers again.

Breastfeeding After a Breast Lift

Most women can breastfeed after a lift.

Some milk ducts are divided during surgery, but many regenerate over time. Temporary pockets of trapped milk can occur and typically resolve on their own.

Some women choose to wait until childbearing is complete. Others prefer to enjoy the benefits now, understanding that a small touch-up may be needed later.

Both choices are valid.

Safety, Blood Flow, and Precision

A breast lift is safe—but not if you smoke or vape.

Nicotine constricts blood vessels and compromises healing, particularly to the nipple. I require complete nicotine abstinence for six weeks before and after surgery. This is what I tell my smoking patients: "Every time you want to light up that cigarette, I want you to look down at your nipples and imagine them turning black and falling off." You must not have any nicotine at all, not even a nicotine patch, an e-cigarette or a "nicotine-free vape"...which still may have small amounts of nicotine.

I will also need to know if you have type 2 diabetes or high blood pressure. These conditions can also cause problems with blood flow to the nipple and can slow down incision healing. If these issues have been addressed and are under control, I can safely operate.

The Breast Lift Procedure

What Actually Happens

A breast lift reshapes tissue, removes excess skin, and elevates the nipple-areolar complex without detaching it.

The most common approach uses an anchor-pattern incision, which allows precise shaping and long-term stability. Scars fade significantly over time and are typically hidden by bras or swimwear.

Surgery takes two to four hours.
Adding augmentation increases time modestly.

In the pre-op area, I draw some markings on your breasts to guide me. "Measure twice, cut once," is my motto. Most women's breasts are naturally a bit asymmetric—one is often a little bit larger than the other. Your surgery can make your breasts match better and get your nipples to line up with one another. But as I tell my patients, "They're sisters, not twins." Our goal is improvement—not perfection.

Recovery and Healing

You'll go home the same day in a supportive bra.

Temporary changes in nipple sensation are common and usually resolve over several months.

Most women:

- Resume light activity within a week
- Return to full activity within two weeks (four weeks if combined with augmentation)

By two months, shape becomes clear.
By four months, the breasts soften into their final, natural contour.

"The Mirror Didn't Surprise Me—It Recognized Me."

Anna stood quietly in front of the mirror at her first post-op visit.

"I didn't gasp," she said.
"I just nodded."

"This feels like alignment," she told me.
"Like my outside finally caught up with my inside."

Results—Over Time

With stable weight and no future pregnancies, breast lift results last many years.

Your breasts will continue to age naturally—but from a stronger, more balanced starting point.

A breast lift does not erase motherhood.
It honors it.

Closing Reflection

A breast lift isn't about becoming someone new.

It's about standing taller in the body that carried you here.

It says:
I gave. I nurtured. I sacrificed.
And now—I choose to restore.

That choice is not vanity.
It is sovereignty.

CHAPTER 20

Heavy, Disproportionate, or Painful? When Breast Reduction is the Right Move

Breast Reduction

Before we talk about cup sizes or incisions, let's talk about weight.
Not the number on the scale—but the kind you carry every day.
The pull on your shoulders.
The ache in your neck.
The way your body leans forward before you even realize it has.

For some women, large breasts are not a feature.
They are a burden quietly carried through motherhood, work, movement, and rest.

If you've ever felt tired before the day even began, this chapter isn't about taking something away.
It's about giving relief back—
to your body,
to your posture,
and sometimes, to your spirit.

When Less Isn't Loss—It's Relief

For some women, breast reduction is not about changing how they look in the mirror. It's about changing how they *feel* in their body.

For many moms, pregnancy and breastfeeding don't just alter breast shape—they amplify what may have already been heavy. It can take what was a small problem and make it bigger, literally. Breasts that were once manageable become uncomfortably large. Supportive bras dig in. Shoulders ache. Backs protest. Skin becomes irritated. Exercise feels impossible. Clothes never quite fit the way you want them to.

And often—quietly, privately—you're tired of carrying the weight.

In these cases, breast reduction (reduction mammoplasty) can be a deeply restorative part of a Mommy Makeover. The procedure allows us to reduce breast size, reshape and rebalance the breasts, restore symmetry, and carefully reposition the nipples into a more natural, youthful position. In many cases, we also address fullness along the bra-strap area or under the arms with liposuction or even direct bra strap excision, smoothing contours that have long felt stubborn and frustrating.

But the most meaningful changes aren't always visible in photos.

They show up in posture.
In comfort.
In movement.
In relief.

Women often tell me they didn't realize just how much their breasts were affecting their daily lives until the burden was gone.

Meet Sarah- The Blonde with "The Chest"

For a decade, she carried a heavy weight—both physically and emotionally. Since she was 14 years old, she had been defined by her body, known simply as "the blonde with the chest." It was a label that overshadowed who she really was.

The physical toll was undeniable. Her chiropractor and other doctors warned her that the weight was actually beginning to curve her spine. Fear of the pain, the cost, and the unknown had held her back for years, but the medical necessity finally pushed her forward. She interviewed four surgeons, but when she met me, she said "I kept telling my husband, I just feel better about Dr. Burgdorf. He just feels right when he looks at me. He understands what I'm hoping for." She felt I truly saw *her*, not just the procedure.

On the day of surgery, the moment of truth came when she got home. Her mother helped her change out of the loose, flowy shirt she used to hide her body. As she stood in front of the mirror in her surgical bra, she burst into tears. For the first time since she was a teenager, she could see her ribcage. It was a profound realization: "That's me." She wasn't wearing compression bras anymore; she was finally at home in her own body. She told me she looks the way she has always seen herself, and now, the world can see her that way too.

More Than Aesthetic Relief

Large, heavy breasts can place real physical strain on the body. Chronic neck, shoulder, and back pain are common. Bra straps leave deep grooves. Rashes and skin breakdown can develop beneath the breasts.

Finding bras that truly fit can feel like a lifelong scavenger hunt—and even then, the support rarely lasts.

Daily activities become more exhausting than they should be. Exercise feels restricted. Clothing choices are limited. And, for some women, unwanted attention or unkind comments add an emotional layer to the physical discomfort.

What many women are surprised to learn is that **even a modest reduction—sometimes just one cup size—can create a meaningful improvement** in comfort, mobility, and quality of life.

Breast reduction isn't about erasing femininity.
It's about restoring balance.

Kathryn – After 18 years, It Was Time for Her

She came to me feeling undeserving, battling the guilt that so many mothers feel when they consider doing something just for themselves. For nearly eighteen years, she had put her children and her husband first. Her body had been through a lot—excessive weight gain during pregnancy, toxemia, and significant stretch marks. One breast was larger than the other, and despite her husband's constant affirmations, she struggled to see her own beauty.

The emotion of the journey nearly stopped her. She almost backed out, overwhelmed by the financial commitment and fear. But on the day of surgery, in the pre-op area, she looked at me and said, "Please make me beautiful." I took her hand and told her, "You are already beautiful. I'm just going to make you more beautiful than you are today."

We performed a breast reduction and lift as part of her transformation. A week later, she was a different person. She told me she loved herself now more than she ever had before. It wasn't just about the physical results; it was about the realization that she was worth the investment.

Breast Reduction Readiness

A Gentle Check-In

If you're considering breast reduction, here are some thoughtful questions to help guide the conversation:

- What have you always wanted your breasts to look and feel like?
- What cup size feels realistic—and comfortable—for *your* body?
- How does your partner feel about a smaller breast size? (If this is a concern, I'm always happy to include them in a conversation focused on health, comfort, and long-term well-being.)
- Have you stopped breastfeeding for at least six months? Your breasts need time to naturally settle before surgery.
- Are you close to a stable, realistic weight for you? While weight changes do affect breast size, women who are naturally well-endowed often cannot diet their way to relief.
- Are you planning future pregnancies? Breastfeeding is usually possible after reduction, but temporary challenges can occur.
- Do you smoke? Smoking must be stopped well before and after surgery to protect healing and nipple circulation.
- Do you have realistic expectations? Reduction can significantly decrease size—but extremely large breasts will likely still be a large size after surgery.

These conversations aren't about qualifying you.
They're about protecting your outcome—and your peace of mind.

"Isn't This the Opposite of a Mommy Makeover?"

It can sound that way at first.

After all, most people associate Mommy Makeovers with adding volume—not removing it. But functionally and surgically, breast reduction is very similar to a breast lift. The difference is simply how much tissue we remove.

The goal is never to make you smaller than your body can safely or naturally support. I've worked with women ranging from F cups to L cups, and sometimes the initial request sounds like, *"Just take them off. I want to be an A."*

While I understand the sentiment, safety matters.

Removing too much tissue can compromise nipple blood flow and create disproportion that doesn't serve your body—or your confidence. My goal is to create breasts that are lighter, lifted, symmetrical, and harmonious with your shoulders, waist, and hips.

Balanced. Natural. Sustainable.

Cup sizes also vary wildly between brands. What one store calls an F, another may label a G. What matters most isn't the letter—it's how your body feels and moves afterward. Once, a patient came in and told me that depending on the store her cup size was E, F, or G. My medical assistant was laughing because she thought I kept referring to this patient's breasts as F'ing G's. I clarified, saying, "Yes, they were large, they were either Fs or G's." In most very large-breasted patients, we can safely reduce into the DD or DDD range while preserving nipple health and long-term results.

One important note: **breast reduction is not weight-loss surgery**. You will weigh a bit less—but the rest of your body remains the same. In fact, once the breasts are lighter, your abdomen may appear more visible simply because it's no longer hidden. This is something we'll discuss openly during planning so there are no surprises.

This isn't about losing part of your body.
It's about releasing what no longer serves you—
and making room for relief.

Insurance Coverage: Proceed with Caution

In some cases, breast reduction *may* qualify for insurance coverage when large breasts cause documented medical problems. Approval, however, is rarely simple. Insurance companies often require extensive proof, such as:

- Repeated visits with a primary care physician or OB/GYN
- Documentation of pain despite supportive bras
- Attempts at conservative treatments like physical therapy or chiropractic care
- Stable weight, with surgery not viewed as a weight-loss solution

Even when approval is granted, coverage often comes with a significant trade-off.

Insurance companies typically dictate *how much* breast tissue must be removed for a reduction to be considered "medically necessary." These formulas are created without ever seeing, meeting, or understanding the woman they affect. They prioritize numbers—not proportions, balance, or long-term appearance.

My responsibility is always to **you**—your body, your goals, and the outcome you'll live with every day. I will recommend a reduction that fits your frame and preserves natural shape, even if it doesn't meet an arbitrary threshold set by someone with no personal relationship to you. I have seen far too many cases where insurance-mandated requirements pushed surgeons toward excessive tissue removal that would have left women misshapen or harmed aesthetically.

Yes, breast reduction is a functional surgery that can relieve pain and improve quality of life. But functional relief should never come at the expense of thoughtful, beautiful results.

Since the first edition of this book was written, insurance requirements have only grown more burdensome — months of documentation, multiple failed therapies, and increasingly unreasonable hurdles (like requirements of hypnosis or acupuncture, as examples) that do nothing to reduce breast size or address the real problem. After watching so many women navigate this exhausting process, I made a deliberate decision to step away from insurance altogether.

By offering care directly, I can focus on what truly matters: doing what is right for *you.* And in many cases, with today's high-deductible plans, patients actually pay less out-of-pocket when bypassing insurance entirely.

My relationship is with you—not an insurance company that never has to meet you, see you, or stand behind the outcome.

The Procedure Itself

Breast reduction surgery typically takes about two to three hours and is performed as an outpatient procedure. It involves removing excess breast tissue and skin, reshaping the remaining tissue, and lifting the nipple-areolar complex while preserving blood flow.

In select cases, liposuction, or even direct bra strap excision, may be used to refine areas near the bra line or under the arms. Larger reductions simply require more time and precision—but the recovery timeline is similar.

Galaflex, a dissolvable mesh, may be offered as a sort of "internal bra" to help support the lower hemisphere of the breast, extending the longevity of the result.

Most patients go home the same day after a brief recovery period.

Recovery & Healing

After surgery, temporary nipple numbness is common, especially with larger reductions. Sensation usually returns gradually over several months, with most women recovering full sensation within a year.

You'll wear a supportive sports bra continuously for the first two weeks, then part-time for another two. Underwire bras should be avoided initially.

Some bruising and minor drainage are normal early on. Wound healing issues are the most common complication, particularly in patients who smoke, have diabetes, or are significantly overweight. When small areas open, they typically heal well with local care and patience.

Pain is usually manageable and short-lived. Once we get below skin level, the remainder of the breast is just fatty tissue and insensate. So, the incisional pain at the skin level is easily managed with a few days of pain medication. Most women return to normal daily activities within 7–10 days, avoiding heavy lifting for about six weeks. There are no drains, and showering is allowed shortly after surgery. Just like with breast lifts, the "hard part" is the waiting game of about four months to see the final shape.

Scar care—including gentle massage and silicone treatments—helps minimize long-term visibility.

Because breast tissue may change after surgery, I require baseline mammograms beforehand and encourage ongoing self-exams. Any new lumps should be evaluated with the understanding that benign changes like fat necrosis can occur and are not cancerous.

Best Birthday Present Ever- To Herself

She treated herself to a breast reduction as a 30th birthday gift, a decision that would pay dividends for years to come. At the time of her surgery, we had open and honest discussions about her future plans to have children and her desire to breastfeed. She needed a surgeon who could preserve that ability while relieving her pain.

Six years later, she is a mother. Her son was born a few years after the surgery, and she was able to breastfeed him successfully. Now expecting her second child, she looks forward to sharing that bonding experience again. Beyond the joys of motherhood, the surgery immediately relieved her back pain and saved her spine from continuing to curve under the weight. When she looks in the mirror now, she sees herself—not simply a "large-chested woman," but a confident person who feels comfortable in her own skin.

The Outcome That Matters Most

Years later, what patients remember most isn't the incision pattern.

It's standing straighter.
Moving freely.
Exercising without pain.
Choosing clothes because they *want* to—not because they have to.

Some women laugh and say, *"I feel so light, I might tip backward."*

Those moments never get old for me.

Because breast reduction isn't about taking something away.
It's about giving comfort back.
And sometimes, that changes everything.

CHAPTER 21
Smaller Adjustments That Make a Big Visual Impact: Bra Strap Excision

The Detail That Changes the Way Everything Fits

Some frustrations don't announce themselves loudly.

They show up in dressing rooms.
In fitted blouses you love from the front—but avoid from the side.
In mirrors that feel unforgiving from behind.

For many women, the area along the bra strap—the soft bulge at the side of the breast, the fold above or below the band, the roll across the upper back—becomes one of the most stubborn reminders of weight change, pregnancy, or simply genetics.

You may work out.
You may eat well.
You may have already addressed your breasts or your abdomen.

And yet, this area lingers.

Bra strap excision exists for exactly this reason.

If you've ever felt finished everywhere *except* here, this chapter is about refinement—not excess.
Not doing more, but finally addressing the detail that never quite resolved on its own.

When Liposuction Isn't the Whole Answer

Many patients come in assuming that these folds are simply excess fat—and that liposuction alone will solve the problem. Occasionally, it helps. But more often, the issue isn't fat.

It's skin.

Skin that has stretched, loosened, and separated slightly from the underlying structures. Skin that no longer snaps back the way it once did. When compressed by a bra, that looseness folds over itself, creating the very bulge you're trying to hide.

In these cases, removing skin—not just fat—creates a far more refined and lasting result.

A bra strap excision allows us to directly remove the excess skin and underlying tissue in the exact pattern where the bra sits, smoothing the upper back, tightening the lateral breast, and restoring continuity to the torso's silhouette.

A Subtle Procedure with Outsized Impact

This is not a surgery most women ask for first.

Often, it's considered after the breasts or abdomen have already been addressed—or once weight loss has stabilized. Sometimes, it becomes unnecessary after a breast lift, augmentation or abdominoplasty. Other times, it's the final detail that completes the transformation.

When combined with a breast lift or reduction, tightening the area from beneath the arm and across the upper back can immediately create the appearance of significant weight loss—because the entire frame begins to look more streamlined from every angle.

This procedure is especially powerful for:

- Women who have experienced massive weight loss
- Mothers with repeated weight fluctuations from pregnancy
- Women who are simply "built this way" and have always carried fullness in the upper trunk

For the right patient, it's not about doing more surgery. It's about finishing well.

This isn't about removing more.
It's about refining what remains—
so the whole silhouette finally feels complete.

Three Ways We Can Address the Bra Strap Area

There are three primary approaches, each with its own role:

1. Liposuction Alone

In my experience, this is often the least effective option. When skin quality is thick or loose, removing fat alone rarely resolves the fold—and can sometimes make the skin look more lax.

2. Liposuction With Skin Tightening (Renuvion)

In select patients, adding Renuvion can tighten the skin by approximately 20–30%. This technology uses radiofrequency energy and helium plasma to contract the fibrous connections beneath the skin, creating a subtle "shrink-wrap" effect.

This can be helpful—but it has limits.

3. Bra Strap Excision (Direct Removal)

This is the most definitive solution. By directly excising excess skin and fat along the bra strap line, we can eliminate the fold entirely and tighten the area in a way no non-excisional method can match.

The tradeoff, of course, is a scar—which leads to the most important conversation of all.

The Honest Tradeoff: Scar for Shape

Bra strap excision involves a linear, elliptical incision across the upper back that may extend toward the sides of the breasts. The incision can be designed to sit within the bra line or angled in a gentle curve—similar to a racerback or "cross-your-heart" bra—depending on how much skin needs to be removed and where you prefer the scar to fall.

The scar is visible without clothing. It may even extend beyond a bikini top coverage. There's really no way around that.

For patients with massive weight loss, this is rarely a deterrent—the relief of losing overhanging skin far outweighs the visibility of a scar. For others, this is a deeply personal decision.

My role is not to convince you.
It's to help you decide whether the exchange is worth it *for you.*

How the Procedure Works

Bra strap excision can be performed alone or combined with other procedures, such as:

- A superior 360° torsoplasty
- Posterior body lift or belt lipectomy
- Breast lift, reduction, or augmentation
- Arm lift (brachioplasty)

The surgery itself is efficient, typically lasting one to two hours. Markings are done with you standing, allowing us to tailor the excision precisely. A simple pinch test determines how much skin can be safely removed while respecting movement and healing.

Drains are usually placed for two to three weeks to prevent fluid accumulation and are typically hidden near the underarm. Because no muscle is involved, pain is generally mild and short-lived—most patients describe a few days of incisional discomfort that responds well to rest and medication.

Overhead reaching and aggressive stretching are restricted for about four weeks to protect the scar as it heals. Scar maturation continues over a year, gradually fading in color and softening in texture.

Why This Can Be a Quietly Life-Changing Choice

For women who choose this surgery thoughtfully and intentionally, the payoff is often emotional as much as physical.

Clothes fit differently—from every angle.
Blouses skim instead of cling.
Tight dresses feel elegant instead of revealing something you wish they wouldn't.

It's not about perfection.

It's about freedom—from adjusting, hiding, layering, and second-guessing.

For the right woman, bra strap excision isn't an "extra" procedure.
It's the final release of something that's been in the way for a very long time.

CHAPTER 22

Labiaplasty and the Art of Intimate Restoration

"Your femininity didn't disappear—it's waiting to be invited back."

There are parts of motherhood we talk about openly.
The sleepless nights.
The stretch marks.
The exhaustion that settles into your bones.

And then there are parts no one seems to talk about—not at dinner, not at church, not even with close friends.

The quiet discomfort.
The subtle pulling, rubbing, or pressure of enlarged labia during an Iron Tribe workout.

The self-consciousness of how you look in your favorite Lululemon leggings.

The moment during intimacy when something feels... *different*.
Not broken. Just unfamiliar. Less responsive. Less *you*.

Many of my patients—doctors, lawyers, and CEOs—admit they felt a sense of guilt even bringing this up. Many women assume this is simply the cost of becoming a mother.

That discomfort is the price of sacrifice.
That silence is a virtue.

It isn't.

Ellie: A Patient Who Became "So Cute Down There"

Ellie was so unhappy with her genital appearance that she just wanted to hide. Being very athletic, she was daily embarrassed about her appearance... in leggings, shorts, yoga pants. During her first post-op appearance, she was beyond thankful. At a month, she was beaming as I entered the clinic room. **"I almost tear up when I look down now! It's just *so cute down there*"**--She says smiling broadly yet all the while holding back tears. She told me she fits better in workout clothes and is so much more confident. Not just while working out, but all the time...it has become a non-issue for her.

After childbirth, many women experience changes in their most intimate anatomy—changes that are physical, emotional, and deeply personal.

The labia—both inner and outer—may become elongated, uneven, or irritated by clothing, exercise, or intimacy.
The clitoral hood can thicken or obscure sensation.

These changes aren't rare.
They aren't shameful.
And they aren't "just cosmetic."

Yet most women carry this quietly.

They avoid certain clothes.
They rush intimacy—or avoid it altogether.
They feel self-conscious in moments meant to be connecting.

Not because they don't love their partner.
Not because they've lost desire.
But because their body no longer feels like a place of ease.

What makes this harder is the guilt layered on top of it.

I should just be grateful.
Other women have it worse.
This feels selfish to even think about.

But here's the truth no one says out loud:

Comfort is not vanity.
Confidence is not indulgence.
Wanting to feel at home in your body again is not weakness—it's self-respect.

This is where **labiaplasty** comes into the conversation—not as taboo procedures, but as thoughtful, restorative options for women who want to feel comfortable, confident, and fully present again.

Intimate restoration is about removing the distractions that keep you from being fully present. When you are no longer worried about discomfort or how you look in the light, the ripple effect on your marriage and your confidence is profound.

Labiaplasty

Labiaplasty focuses on the external anatomy—the labia minora, labia majora, and sometimes the clitoral hood.

For some women, the concern is appearance. For others, it's physical discomfort during exercise, intimacy, or daily movement. Often, it's both.

Hormonal changes, childbirth, and genetics can all contribute to elongation or asymmetry. Labiaplasty reshapes and refines this tissue with artistry and restraint—never excessive, never aggressive.

The goal is **natural, balanced, and unrecognizable as "surgery."** Just comfort. Ease. Confidence.

As a plastic surgeon, I approach this with an eye for symmetry and natural beauty that a general gynecologist simply isn't trained to see. My goal is by hiding incisions in natural creases and using dissolving sutures, the only thing people notice (including your partner) is your renewed radiance.

Many women are hesitant to bring this up—especially with a male surgeon. I understand that hesitation deeply. My role is not to judge or rush, but to create a space where *nothing about your body is awkward or off-limits.* If it matters to you, it matters.

That is why I've designed my consultation to be a sanctuary of privacy and respect. We wait until you are fully healed from childbirth (at least six months) to ensure we are working with your body's true "new normal." From the "peri bottle" self-care rituals you remember from your first days of motherhood to the gentle follow-up care my Nashville team provides, you are protected every step of the way.

With today's trend of close grooming in the genital area, many women are very much aware of their appearance and want to do something about it. Labiaplasty (even for women who have never had children) has become much more popular in the past couple of decades.

Hormonal changes during pregnancy, combined with childbirth, can enlarge and stretch out the internal and external labia and the clitoral hood. The labia are now bigger and may also be uneven in size and shape. I want you to wait a minimum of three to six months after childbirth before doing a labiaplasty so the swelling is resolved and the healing is complete. If you experienced any tears or trauma during delivery, I want all to be back to normal before we even consider labiaplasty.

Many women start life with naturally asymmetric labia—they're just born that way, but childbirth can make the problem worse. The clitoral hood can become larger and thicker and covers more of the clitoris.

All this can make a mom feel very self-conscious about her intimate appearance. Enlarged labia can make intercourse physically uncomfortable and also cause discomfort when you're working out or wearing tight-fitting clothing (think swimsuit, yoga pants or skinny jeans). An enlarged clitoral hood can decrease sensation when having sex. Labiaplasty can decrease and reconfigure the shape of the vaginal lips and help restore the area to a more youthful and attractive state.

Labiaplasty has three major components:

- Labia Majora Reduction
- Labia Minora Reduction
- Clitoral Hood Reduction

How These Procedures Are Performed

These procedures can be part of a Mommy Makeover or done separately (or individually) as outpatient surgery under local anesthetic with a blood constrictor to minimize pain and bleeding. The procedure, in any form, takes only about an hour.

To reduce and reshape the labia, I remove an asymmetric, wedge-shaped portion of the tissue and then suture the remaining tissue into a natural shape. I will not only reduce the size of the labia, I will make them more even and symmetric. I will also remove any excess tissue in the clitoral hood area.

I carefully orient the incisions so that scarring doesn't cause problems as the area heals. I don't want the vaginal opening to get tighter or to pull on the internal vaginal tissue. I use dissolving sutures to hold everything together. Most of the scarring will be invisible inside the vaginal tunnel. I hide the external incisions in the natural creases of the area; they usually fade away quickly anyway. If the clitoral hood is covered up, I can extend the incision or make a separate incision to expose the clitoris a bit more. While many women find this increases their enjoyment of sex, I am very careful not to remove too much in this area. Overstimulation can be more uncomfortable than enjoyable. And we need to ensure that the clitoris is still protected and doesn't get irritated.

Precision here is not optional; it is essential.

This is not a place for shortcuts.
It's a place for experience, respect, and restraint.

After The Surgery

Despite how intimidating surgery in this area *sounds*, recovery is usually far gentler than expected.

Most of my patients who do it separately from their Mommy Makeover need very little pain medication and are back to their usual activities quickly. Swelling and soreness are common early on. Because the area is much like the inside of your mouth, it heals quickly, just as a small cut inside your cheek does.

You'll recognize some of the postpartum care routines: gentle rinsing, protective measures, time. We will send you home with a handheld squirt bottle (peri bottle) to rinse yourself after you urinate and when you are showering. Be very gentle at first. Use the bottle for about a week until the incisions are healed.

Labiaplasty is generally very, very safe. Infection, bleeding, and an overabundance of scar tissue are rare complications. Should you develop a hematoma (a bit of pooled blood) in the area, it could swell and be painful, but it isn't dangerous—and it's easy to treat, so please call me right away.

For the first month or so after the surgery, you will need to avoid using tampons; pads are fine. To avoid infection, skip baths, hot tubs, and swimming for three weeks. We do recommend sitz baths after each bowel movement during this healing period to ensure the area is cleaned well. And no intercourse for four to six weeks until you are completely healed.

Your new appearance shouldn't change over time or even with more children. As always, it's a good idea to avoid excessive weight gain or loss.

You aren't just "fixing a problem." You are reclaiming a part of yourself that was set aside. You are choosing to be the "Super Mom" who also feels like a "Super Woman"

And the results?

They don't announce themselves.
They simply *feel right.*

Comfort in clothing.
Ease in movement.
Presence during intimacy.

And perhaps most importantly—relief from carrying something silently for years.

Briana- No Adjustment Needed Anymore!

"Labiaplasty is the best thing I've ever done. It is awesome. I didn't realize how uncomfortable it was before getting surgery and now it is the best. My clothes fit better, leggings are better, underwear is better, there's no adjustment needing to be made throughout the day. I think every mom needs to do it. It's amazing. It's so worth it. It's so comfortable... Makes you feel better as a new mom, I think. I'm just your average mom, I stay home with the kids, we run around with the kids and the recovery has been great. I feel really good. I'm so happy. Don't be afraid to get it done. It's the best thing ever! It's life changing!"

The Deeper Truth

For many women, this isn't just about anatomy.

It's about reclaiming a part of themselves that quietly stepped aside during years of caregiving.

It's about no longer apologizing—to themselves or anyone else—for wanting to feel whole.

When confidence is restored privately, it has a way of rippling outward—into relationships, presence, and how a woman carries herself in the world.

That ripple matters.

Activity: A Private Moment With Yourself

Take a few quiet minutes—just for you.

In a journal, or even in the notes app on your phone, write honestly:

"If I were 100% comfortable in my own skin—if the physical irritation and the mental self-consciousness were simply gone—how would I show up differently in my most intimate relationships?"

Would intimacy feel different?
Would movement feel freer?
Would you stop editing yourself in quiet moments?

There is no right answer.
Only your answer.

And you are allowed to listen to it.

Visualize that version of you. She is still there. She is just waiting for the invitation to return.

CHAPTER 23
Becoming Visible Again

"Learning to receive the woman you've become."

There is a quiet moment that comes after the healing.

Not the physical healing—that comes first.

The swelling fades. The incisions soften. The mirror becomes less intimidating.

But then something more subtle happens.

You are seen.

A compliment lands.
A glance lingers.
Someone says, *"You look amazing,"* and instead of absorbing it, your instinct is to deflect:

"Oh, it's just the lighting."
"I've just been trying to eat better."
"It's nothing, really."

For many mothers, this is the unexpected part.

Not the surgery.
Not the recovery.

But the **visibility**.

The Habit of Disappearing

Motherhood, in many ways, teaches women how to disappear.

Not entirely—but incrementally.

You become the one who organizes, supports, anticipates, absorbs.
You learn to meet everyone else's needs before your own.
You become fluent in selflessness.

And over time, something subtle shifts:

You stop expecting to be seen.

So when visibility returns—whether through confidence, posture, presence, or physical change—it can feel unfamiliar. Even uncomfortable.

Not because it's wrong.
But because it's been absent.

Receiving Without Explaining

There is a difference between being seen...
and allowing yourself to be seen.

The first happens automatically.
The second is a practice.

When someone offers a compliment, what they are really offering is acknowledgment:

I see you.
I notice the change.
I recognize something in you.

And the simplest, most powerful response is often the hardest:

"Thank you."

Not followed by an explanation.
Not softened with dismissal.
Not redirected.

Just received.

Embodiment: Living Inside the Change

Transformation is not complete when the procedure is done.
It is complete when the identity catches up.

That means learning to:

- Stand differently
- Walk differently
- Dress with intention instead of apology
- Make eye contact without shrinking
- Accept space instead of minimizing your presence

This is not performance.
It is embodiment.

And it takes practice.

Confidence Ritual

For the next week, notice every time someone offers you praise.

Instead of deflecting, try this:

- Pause
- Breathe
- Say, **"Thank you"**
- Let it land

That's it.

You are not learning how to become someone new.
You are learning how to **receive who you already are**.

A Different Kind of Strength

There is strength in sacrifice.
Every mother knows that.

But there is also strength in presence.
In visibility.
In allowing yourself to be fully expressed without apology.

You didn't vanish.
You adapted.

And now—you're returning.

Not to who you were before.

But to someone more aware, more grounded, more fully yourself.

CHAPTER 24
The Ripple Effect
How One Woman's Confidence Changes Everything Around Her

"When a mom's confidence rises, her whole family stands taller."

Confidence is rarely contained.

It doesn't stay neatly within the boundaries of one person.

It moves.

It echoes.

It spreads.

Especially in a family.

The Misconception of "Selfish"

Many women hesitate before doing something for themselves—not because they don't want it, but because they worry about what it means.

Is this selfish?
Is this necessary?
Shouldn't I be focusing on everyone else?

But what often goes unseen is this:

When a mother reconnects with herself, everyone around her benefits.

Not because she becomes different—
but because she becomes **more present**.

What Changes First

The changes are rarely dramatic at first.

They show up in small ways:

- A little more patience
- A little less irritation
- A willingness to be in photos instead of behind the camera
- More eye contact
- More laughter

Children notice.
Partners notice.
Even if they can't name it.

What they are responding to is **ease**.

The Emotional Tone of a Home

Every home has an emotional tone.

It's shaped not by perfection—but by presence.

When a mother feels depleted, stretched thin, or disconnected from herself, that tone shifts. Subtly, but consistently.

And when she feels grounded—when she feels like herself again—that tone shifts back.

Not louder.
Not forced.

Just steadier.

Modeling Without Saying a Word

Children learn more from what we embody than what we explain.

When they see a mother who:

- Takes care of herself without guilt
- Accepts compliments without deflection
- Shows up with confidence instead of apology

They internalize something powerful:

This is what it looks like to value yourself.

And that lesson lasts far longer than anything spoken at the dinner table.

Family Gratitude Moment

This week, try something simple.

At dinner, ask each person to share:

- One thing they're proud of
- One thing they appreciate about someone else at the table

Keep it short. Keep it light.

You may be surprised what surfaces.

The Marriage Shift

Confidence changes the dynamic of a relationship—not through pressure, but through presence.

When a woman feels more at home in her body:

- Communication softens
- Physical connection becomes more natural
- Playfulness returns

It's not about becoming someone different for your partner.

It's about removing the quiet barriers that distance creates.

The Ripple You Didn't Expect

Most women come in thinking about one outcome:

"I just want to feel better about myself."

What they don't expect is everything that follows:

- Saying yes more easily
- Showing up more fully
- Feeling less reactive, more grounded
- Being seen—and allowing it

Confidence, when it's real, doesn't stay contained.

It becomes part of the environment.

And everyone feels it.

Afterword
The Woman in the Mirror

"You didn't go back—you went forward."

There is a moment—quiet, almost easy to miss—
when everything settles.

The appointments are behind you.
The healing has softened.
The mirror no longer feels like something to evaluate.

And then, one day, you look...
and you recognize her.

Not perfectly.
Not dramatically.

But honestly.

This was never about becoming someone new.

It was about remembering.
Reclaiming.
Allowing yourself to take up space again—without apology.

If you've made it here, you've already done something meaningful:

You paused.
You reflected.
You considered yourself.

That alone is powerful.

If there is one thing I hope you carry forward, it's this:

You are allowed to feel at home in your body.
You are allowed to want more for yourself.
You are allowed to be seen.

Not later.
Not after everything else is done.

Now.

And when you catch your reflection again—
in a mirror, a window, a passing moment—

I hope you don't analyze what you see.

I hope you recognize it.

And if, as you close this book, someone comes to mind—
a woman who is quietly carrying more than she shows...
a woman who has learned to put herself last...
a woman who might need this reminder more than she realizes—

Trust that instinct.

For the Woman You're Thinking Of

There's a reason this book is in your hands.

And there may be someone else who needs it too.

Not because she's "ready."
Not because she's asked.

But because she's been quietly putting herself last.

Write Her a Note

Dear____

Here's what I want you to know:

____

____

____

____

____

____

With Love, ____

Sometimes the most powerful message isn't in the book—
it's the one that says, **"I see you."**

About the Author Page

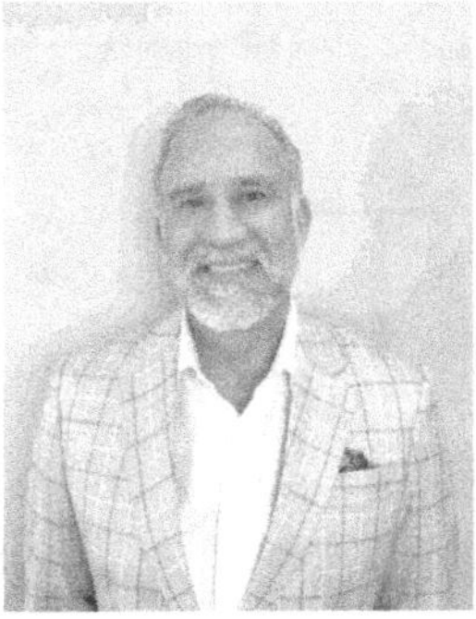

Michael R. Burgdorf, MD, MPH is a board-certified plastic surgeon, nationally recognized author, and the founder of Music City Plastic Surgery in Nashville, Tennessee — where he has spent more than fifteen years helping women restore not just their appearance, but their relationship with themselves.

Known by his patients as *The Gentleman Surgeon*, Dr. Burgdorf is celebrated for his meticulous artistry, exceptional bedside manner, and his signature aesthetic — the Nashville Natural — results that are balanced, proportional, and beautifully precise without ever looking overdone. He was certified by the American Board of Plastic Surgery in 2011 and has been recognized as a Top 10 Plastic Surgeon in Tennessee by the American Institute of Plastic Surgeons every year since — a distinction held by fewer than ten physicians in the state.

Dr. Burgdorf is a two-time Amazon number-one bestselling author. His first book, *The Mommy Makeover: Restoring Your Body After Childbirth* (Advantage Media Group, 2015), simultaneously reached number one in Plastic Surgery, Plastic Cosmetic Surgery, and Hot New Releases on Amazon — and also earned a Mom's Choice Silver Award, placing second overall behind Pampers and making him the only physician in the award's history to receive that honor. His second book, *The Daddy Do-Over: Boost Your Confidence in the Boardroom and the Bedroom* (Advantage Media Group, 2018), also reached number one on Amazon. This volume — *The Mommy Makeover: How Real Moms Reclaim Confidence, Connection, and Their Reflection* — is his most personal work to date.

The recipient of more than a dozen regional and national awards — including the Doctor's Choice Award, voted by fellow physicians, the Patient's Choice Award, the Most Compassionate Doctor Award, and recognition as a Top 1% Most Honored Professional in America — Dr. Burgdorf has been consistently recognized by both patients and peers throughout his career. He was inducted into the Gold Humanism Honor Society in medical school, an honor reserved for physicians who demonstrate exceptional compassion, integrity, and service. He is also a RealSelf Top Doctor, the platform's highest designation for surgeons.

Dr. Burgdorf earned his Medical Degree and Master of Public Health simultaneously at Tulane University, where he also began his General Surgery residency. When Hurricane Katrina devastated New Orleans, his residency was interrupted. He continued and completed his General Surgery training at the University of Mississippi Medical Center, where he subsequently completed his residency in Plastic and Reconstructive Surgery.

Before medicine, he was a linebacker at the University of Notre Dame — where the discipline of the game quietly shaped the precision and composure he brings to the operating room today. His most important accomplishment, however, is his marriage of more than twenty-five years to his wife, Casey, and the lives of their four children. An avid college football fan, he enjoys fine wine, good food, and the remarkable lifestyle of the Nashville area, where he and his family are proud to call home.

His consultations are widely regarded as the most comprehensive in Nashville — and possibly the country — featuring his proprietary 5-Star Breast Sizing System and 6-String Assessment, designed to ensure every patient achieves her ideal result through the Goldilocks Phenomenon: not too much, not too little — just right, for her. His follow-up process spans more than a full year, because in his view, the relationship doesn't end when surgery does.

Dr. Burgdorf has been featured on HLN's *Morning Express*, *The Doctors*, and quoted in *The Wall Street Journal*, *The Week*, *Fox News.com*, and *Haute Living*, and has been interviewed on international radio. All procedures are performed at Nashville South Surgery Center — his private, state-of-the-art facility designed for the highest standards of safety, luxury, and privacy.

He wrote this book because he kept seeing the same thing across his consultation table: brilliant, devoted mothers who had quietly stopped seeing themselves. Women who had placed their own confidence on a shelf labeled *Someday* — and needed someone to finally say: *Someday can be now.*

Because he believes that when one woman reclaims her confidence, that ripple touches everyone around her.

Music City Plastic Surgery — Nashville, Tennessee

musiccityplasticsurgery.com

Instagram: @musiccityplasticsurgery

www.ingramcontent.com/pod-product-compliance
Lightning Source LLC
La Vergne TN
LVHW022200200926
848481LV00006B/1796
9798996189816